# MILADY'S STANDARD
# Nail Technology Workbook

*Fifth Edition*

**Milady's Standard Nail Technology Student Workbook**
**Compiled by Jeryl Geary**

COPYRIGHT © 2008 Milady,
a part of Cengage Learning, Inc.

Printed in United States
1 2 3 4 5 XXX 11 10 09 08 07

For more information contact Milady,
a part of Cengage Learning, Inc.
5 Maxwell Drive, Clifton Park, NY 12065–2919.

Or you can visit our Internet site at
http://www.milady.com.

Library of Congress Cataloging-in-Publication Data
ISBN 13: 9781428359499
ISBN 10: 1-4283-5949-4

## NOTICE TO THE READER

Publisher does not warrant or guarantee any of the products described herein or perform any independent analysis in connection with any of the product information contained herein. Publisher does not assume, and expressly disclaims, any obligation to obtain and include information other than that provided to it by the manufacturer.

The reader is expressly warned to consider and adopt all safety precautions that might be indicated by the activities herein and to avoid all potential hazards. By following the instructions contained herein, the reader willingly assumes all risks in connection with such instructions.

The Publisher makes no representation or warranties of any kind, including but not limited to, the warranties of fitness for particular purpose or merchantability, nor are any such representations implied with respect to the material set forth herein, and the publisher takes no responsibility with respect to such material. The Publisher shall not be liable for any special, consequential, or exemplary damages resulting, in whole or part, from the readers' use of, or reliance upon, this material.

# Contents

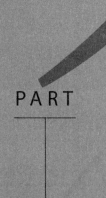

PART

# ORIENTATION

# History and Opportunities

## INTRODUCTION

1. Cosmetology comes from the Greek word *kosmetikos,* meaning _____.

2. List the three broad areas covered by cosmetology.

   a. _____

   b. _____

   c. _____

3. Which was the first known society to cultivate beauty in an extravagant fashion? _____

4. Name the seven natural ingredients that ancient people use as coloring matter on their hair, skin and nails.

   a. _____

   b. _____

   c. _____

   d. _____

   e. _____

   f. _____

   g. _____

5. Women in ancient Greece used _____ on their faces, _____ on their eyes, and ground _____ on their cheeks.

6. Aristocrats in China were known to _____ their nails as early as _____.

7. What mixture of materials did the Chinese aristocrats use to color their nails?

   a. _____

   b. _____

   c. _____

   d. _____

8. In 1400 BC, Nefertiti used _____ to _____ her nails.

9. Charles Revson invented _____ in the early 1930s.

10. The idea for nail lacquer came from which industry? _____

## SALON MANAGEMENT

11. As a licensed nail technician, management opportunities include:

    a. _____

    b. _____

    c. _____

    d. _____

    e. _____

    f. _____

    g. _____

12. Career opportunities outside the salon include:

    a. _____

    b. _____

    c. _____

    d. _____

    e. _____

13. What are the three basic salon business models that employ nail technicians?

    a. _____

    b. _____

    c. _____

14. List four things you can do every day that will put you one step closer to your goal of becoming a successful nail technician:

    a. _____

    b. _____

    c. _____

    d. _____

## MATCHING REVIEW

*Insert the correct word or term in front of each definition.*

Juliet wraps                    Jeff Pink                    full-service salon
kosmetikos                      cosmetology

15. _____ Greek word meaning "skilled in the use of cosmetics"

16. _____ the first paper nail wrapping system

17. _____ offering hair, skin, and nail services

18. _____ beautifying and improving the nails, skin, and hair

19. _____ credited with creating ridge filler and fiber nail strengtheners

# Life Skills

## INTRODUCTION

1. Having great life skills makes it easier to _____ for your entire career.

2. The salon is a highly _____ atmosphere that requires strong _____ and excellent _____.

3. No matter how you feel, or how many hours you have already worked on a given day, you must greet every client with _____.

4. Describe the life skills that can lead to a more satisfying and successful career:

    a. Being genuinely _____ and _____

    b. Readily _____ to different situations

    c. Seeing jobs through to _____

    d. Being _____ with your work

    e. Developing and practicing _____

    f. Making good _____

    g. Feeling good about _____

    h. Being _____

    i. Defining and living by your own _____

    j. Having a strong sense of _____ toward your _____

    k. Being _____

    l. Maintaining a _____

    m. Practicing _____

    n. Striving for _____

5. To be successful, you must take ownership of your education and your career. What does this mean?

    _____

6. List at least seven rules or habits practiced by successful students:

    a. _____

    b. _____

    c. _____

d. _____

e. _____

f. _____

g. _____

h. _____

i. _____

7. What ten guiding principles will help turn the possibilities in your life into realities?

   a. Having good _____

   b. Always _____ your goals

   c. Building on your _____

   d. Being good to _____

   e. Defining your own _____

   f. Practicing positive _____

   g. Separating your _____ and _____ lives

   h. Investing your _____ wisely

   i. _____ others

   j. Staying _____

8. Define procrastination. _____

9. Define perfectionism. _____

10. Define game plan. _____

11. Name the two types of goals: _____ and _____ .

12. You can enhance your creativity in the workplace by:

   a. _____

   b. _____

   c. _____

   d. _____

## MANAGING YOUR CAREER

13. Every successful business has what kind of plan? _____

14. An essential part of this plan is a _____ that establishes the

   _____ of the business, as well as _____ .

15. In one or two sentences, your personal mission statement should communicate

   _____ and _____ .

16. Write down your own personal mission statement. _____

    _____

17. How often should you read your mission statement? _____

## GOAL SETTING

18. Why should you practice goal setting? _____

19. Name two basic types of goals: _____.

20. Short-term goals are those you want to accomplish in what amount of time? _____

21. Long-term goals are those you want to accomplish in what amount of time? _____

## TIME MANAGEMENT

22. How should you prioritize your tasks? _____

    _____

23. You should customize your own time management system by taking into account your

    _____.

24. By listening to your inner organizer, you can identify the times of the day when you are

    _____, and when you _____.

25. If you need a fair amount of flexibility in your schedule, you can stay on top of your tasks by

    _____.

26. Time management also means never taking on more than _____, by learning to say

    _____ firmly, but kindly.

27. Any time you feel frustrated, overwhelmed, or overly worried, you should give yourself some

    _____.

28. Exercise and recreation stimulate _____ and _____.

29. To keep on track, schedule at least one additional block of _____ each day to

    handle _____.

30. List the five key questions you must ask yourself when creating a goal-setting plan.

    a. _____

    b. _____

    c. _____

    d. _____

    e. _____

## STUDY SKILLS

31. Any time studying seems to be overwhelming, you should _____.

32. Where should you study? _____

## ETHICS

33. Define "ethics." _____

34. Each state board of cosmetology sets the ethical standards for _____ and
    _____ that all nail technicians must follow while working in a salon.

35. Important professional ethics include:

    a. _____

    b. _____

    c. _____

    d. _____

36. Define the seven elements of a well-developed attitude.

    a. Diplomacy is _____.

    b. Emotional stability means _____.

    c. Sensitivity is _____.

    d. Values _____; goals _____.

    e. Receptivity involves _____.

    f. Communication skills allow us to _____.

    g. Tone of voice lets you _____.

## MATCHING REVIEW

*Insert the correct word or term to the left of each definition.*

| | | |
|---|---|---|
| ethics | game plan | goal-setting |
| mission statement | perfectionism | prioritize |
| procrastination | self-esteem | motivation |
| self-management | integrity | |

37. _____ arrange a list of tasks in the order of importance

38. _____ making sure your behavior match your actions

39. _____ an organization's purpose, business philosophy and future goals

40. _____ instinctively propels you to do something

41. _____ trusting your ability to reach your goals

42. _____ a set of moral principles or values

43. _____ putting off an action to a later time

44. _____ a well thought out process for the long haul

45. _____ helps you to decide what you want out of life

46. _____ anything less than flawless is unacceptable

47. _____ planning your life, rather than just letting things happen

Date _____

Rating _____

Text Pages 26–33

# Your Professional Image

## INTRODUCTION

1. Why is your future success in the image industry dependent on how well you are groomed, as well as the caliber of your technical skills? _____

_____

## BEAUTY AND WELLNESS
### *Personal Hygiene*

2. Define personal hygiene. _____

_____

3. If you offend clients by having body odor or appearing unkempt, what are they most likely to do? (*Circle the correct answer.*)

   a. Tell you that you have bad body odor or soiled clothing.

   b. Say nothing, but still return to you because you are a skilled nail technician.

   c. Say nothing, but find another nail technician to take care of their beauty needs.

4. What is a hygiene pack? _____

_____.

5. List six things that should be included in your hygiene pack:

   a. _____

   b. _____

   c. _____

   d. _____

   e. _____

   f. _____

6. If you smoke a cigarette, what are the three most important things you must do before servicing a client?

   a. _____

   b. _____

   c. _____

## Looking Good

7. An extremely important element of your image is having well-groomed hair, skin, and nails that serve:

   _____

8. In addition to reflecting current fashions, what must you do to keep your hair, skin, and nails looking their best?

   a. _____

   b. _____

   c. _____

## Fragrance

9. In a salon setting you should: (*Circle the correct answer.*)

   a. Avoid wearing perfume at work.

   b. Keep perfume usage to a minimum.

   c. Wear perfume when and where you like.

## Personal Grooming

10. In terms of personal hygiene, clothing should be: _____ and _____.

# DRESS FOR SUCCESS

11. To ensure that you are in sync with your work environment, your clothing choices should: (*Circle the best answer.*)

    a. Represent the latest fashions

    b. Reflect the personality of the salon

    c. Flatter your figure

12. While you will always be guided by your salon's dress code, list four general wardrobe guidelines:

    a. _____

    b. _____

    c. _____

    d. _____

## The Art of Makeup

13. Describe how your makeup should be in tune with both your personal style and the personality of your salon: _____

    _____

    _____

## YOUR PHYSICAL PRESENTATION

14. Good posture is a very important part of your physical presentation. Name the five ways you can practice good posture at work:

    a. Keep your neck _____ and _____ directly above the _____.

    b. Lift your _____ so that your _____ is out and up.

    c. Hold your shoulders _____ and _____.

    d. Sit with your back _____.

    e. Pull in your _____.

## ERGONOMICS

15. Each year, hundreds of nail technicians develop carpal tunnel syndrome and back injuries. These injuries are called _____.

16. An awareness of your body posture and movements, coupled with _____ and proper _____ will enhance your health and comfort.

17. Define ergonomics. _____

    _____

18. Stressful repetitive motions have a _____ effect on the muscles and joints. Describe the ways that you can prevent repetitive motion injuries:

    a. Use _____ designed implements.

    b. Never _____ or _____ implements too tightly.

    c. Avoid constantly _____ the wrist when using manicuring tools.

    d. Make sure that your _____ are never more than _____ away from your body for extended periods of time.

    e. Never _____ to get closer to your clients. Ask them to _____ their arms or legs _____ to you.

## MATCHING REVEW

*Insert the correct word or term at the left of each definition.*

ergonomics                  dress code                    professional image

physical presentation       musculoskeletal disorders     salon personality

19. _____ set of rules set forth by a business that specify the correct manner of dress

20. _____ the impression you project in the workplace

21. _____ physical injuries caused by performing unsafe manual tasks

22. _____ the style and business focus of the salon

23. _____ changing the work environment to meet the physical needs of workers

24. _____ your posture, gait, and overall body movements

Date _____

Rating _____

Text Pages 34–54

# Communicating for Success

## INTRODUCTION

1. In order to have a thriving beauty career, you must have good _____, _____, and _____ skills.

2. The best way to understand others is to first have a firm understanding of _____.

3. The following are good ways to handle the ups and downs of relationships:

   a. Respond instead of _____.

   b. Believe in _____.

   c. Talk _____, listen _____.

   d. Be _____.

   e. Take your own _____.

4. Human relations can be _____ or _____, depending on how willing you are to give.

5. Complete the following golden rules of human relations:

   a. Communicate from your heart; _____.

   b. A _____ is far more valuable than a _____.

   c. It is easy to make a(n) _____; it is harder to keep a(n) _____.

   d. Ask for _____ instead of just _____.

   e. Show people you care by _____.

   f. Tell people how _____ they are, even if they're not _____.

   g. Being _____ is different from acting _____.

   h. For every _____ you do for others, do something for _____.

   i. _____ often.

   j. Show _____ with other people's flaws.

   k. Build shared _____.

   j. _____ is the best relationship builder.

## COMMUNICATION BASICS

6. Define communication. _____

_____

7. People communicate through _____, _____, _____, _____, and _____.

8. A client intake form should be filled out by every _____ prior to receiving _____.

9. What is a client consultation? _____

   _____

10. Describe a classic look. _____

11. Describe a dramatic look. _____

12. List four things that you need to know about your client's lifestyle before beginning a service.

    a.  _____

    b.  _____

    c.  _____

    d.  _____

13. After you have gathered all the information that you feel you need to understand what your client is saying, you should still _____ this information, using different words and pictures or drawings. This is called _____.

14. If a tardy client arrives and you have time to take care of her without making subsequent clients late for their appointments, you should: (*Circle the best answer.*)

    a.  Let her know that you can take her this time, even though she is late.

    b.  Tell her you cannot take her, even if you have time, to teach her a lesson.

    c.  Let her know you can still do her nails because you have a break after her scheduled appointment, even though she is late.

15. You are running 20 minutes late with your current client and Mrs. Smith will be there shortly. How should you handle this situation? List the three most important steps you should take to keep Mrs. Smith happy.

    a.  _____

    b.  _____

    c.  _____

16. List six important things you should do when dealing with an unhappy client:

    a.  Never _____.

    b.  Ask for _____ about why she is _____.

    c.  If you can make her happy, _____.

    d.  If you cannot make her happy on the spot, _____.

    e.  Offer to _____ the situation _____.

    f.  If the client is still unhappy, _____.

17. Even though clients may think of you as a friend, it is important to always maintain a

_____. Your sole responsibility is to _____.

18. List seven things that describe professional salon behavior.

a. _____

b. _____

c. _____

d. _____

e. _____

f. _____

g. _____

19. The best thing to do is to try to _____ the decisions and rules the manager makes, whether you

agree with them or not.

20. The manager's job is to ensure the salon is _____, and not to deal with technicians'

_____.

21. Before approaching the manager about a work-related problem, you should first come up with possible

_____.

22. Salons that are well run will make it a priority to conduct frequent and thorough _____.

## MATCHING REVIEW

*Insert the correct word or term at the left of each definition.*

reflective listening          client consultation          communication

intake form          employee evaluation          life skills

23. _____ performance review

24. _____ accurate exchange of information by means of speaking, writing, and/or

using visual aids

25. _____ ability to build sound, harmonious relationships with self, others, and the

environment

26. _____ repeating back information to a client, using different words or signs to

ensure that you clearly understand what they are saying

27. _____ verbal communication between a service provider and a client to determine

the desired results

28. _____ client questionnaire that asks for contact information, past history with beauty

services, and any related health or lifestyle issues that would be contraindicative of having a nail service

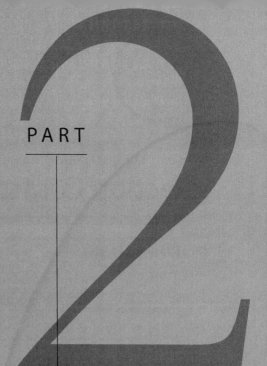

PART

# GENERAL SCIENCES

Date _____

Rating _____

Text Pages 56–85

# Infection Control: Principles and Practice

## INTRODUCTION

1.  Why do regulatory agencies and governmental health departments require that all nail technicians follow certain sanitation procedures? _____

    _____

    _____

## BACTERIA

2.  What are bacteria? Are all bacteria harmful? _____

    _____

3.  What is the difference between nonpathogenic and pathogenic bacteria? _____

    _____

4.  List the three types of pathogenic bacteria discussed in this chapter.

    a. _____ Short rod-shaped bacteria

    b. _____ Round-shaped bacteria

    c. _____ Spiral or corkscrew-shaped bacteria.

5.  What are the most common type of bacteria? _____

6.  Cocci can appear singly or in groups. Name and describe these groups.

    a. _____

    b. _____

    c. _____

7.  **Identification.** Using the letters **A**, **B**, **C**, **D**, and **E** (defined below), match the correct disease characteristics listed below with one type of pathogenic bacteria.

    **Key:**                      **Characteristics:**

    **A**=staphylococci           _____ 1. blood poisoning

    **B**=streptococci            _____ 2. tuberculosis

    **C**=diplococci              _____ 3. syphilis

    **D**=bacilli                 _____ 4. abscesses

    **E**=spirilla                _____ 5. diphtheria

_____ 6. pneumonia

_____ 7. boils

_____ 8. strep throat

_____ 9. tetanus (lockjaw)

_____ 10. toxic shock syndrome

_____ 11. pustules

_____ 12. Lyme disease

_____ 13. typhoid fever

_____ 14. food poisoning

8. Some bacteria are capable of _____ or self-movement; other bacteria are transmitted through the air on _____ or within the substance in which they settle.

9. _____ and _____ are both motile, and use hair-like extensions called _____ or _____ to move about.

10. During the active stage, bacteria thrive in _____, _____, _____, and _____ places.

11. When bacteria reach a certain size, they divide into two new cells called _____. This process is called _____.

12. What is a local infection? _____

_____

13. Another word for contagious is _____.

14. Name nine ways that bacteria and viruses can be spread in a salon situation.

a. _____

b. _____

c. _____

d. _____

e. _____

f. _____

g. _____

h. _____

i. _____

15. Define virus. _____

16. How do viruses live? _____

17. _____ are disease-causing bacteria or viruses that are carried through the body in the _____ or _____. Examples include _____

18. HIV is the virus that causes _____ or _____. AIDS is a _____ that breaks down the body's _____.

19. What should you tell a client who expresses concern about contracting HIV as the result of a nail service? _____

_____

_____

## PARASITES

20. What is a parasite? _____

21. Fungi are parasites that include _____, _____, and _____, that can produce _____ diseases.

22. Nail fungus can be caused by improperly disinfected _____, or when the _____ nail has been improperly treated before an _____ is applied.

23. During a nail service, pathogens can enter the body through:

    a. _____

    b. _____

    c. _____

    d. _____

    e. _____

24. The two types of immunity are _____ and _____.

25. Define decontamination. _____

26. From most- to least-effective, list the three steps of decontamination.

    a. _____

    b. _____

    c. _____

27. Define sterilization. _____

28. Define disinfection. _____

29. Define sanitation. _____

30. The Occupational Safety and Health Administration (OSHA) requires manufacturers to provide a Material Safety Data Sheet (MSDS) for all products used in the salon. List six important things included on an MSDS.

    a. _____

    b. _____

    c. _____

d. _____

e. _____

f. _____

31. In a salon setting, disinfectants must be _____, _____ and _____.

32. All nail implements must be _____ before being submerged in a

_____ to avoid _____ the solution.

33. Any time a nail implement comes in contact with blood or body fluids, it should be

_____.

34. Name four types of disinfectants that are used in salons.

a. _____

b. _____

c. _____

d. _____

35. In the salon, to be effective, the concentration of ethyl and isopropyl alcohol solutions must be no less

than _____%.

36. Disinfectants are powerful products. If used incorrectly, they can be _____. List nine

safety tips that you should follow when handling disinfectants.

a. When mixing, always _____.

b. Always add disinfectant _____; not _____.

c. To remove implements from disinfectants, use _____.

d. Always keep disinfectants out of the _____.

e. Never pour disinfectant _____. If you get disinfectants on your skin,

immediately _____.

f. Carefully _____ all products according to label instructions.

g. Never place any disinfectant in _____.

h. Always follow the _____ for mixing, using, and disposal of disinfectants.

i. Change disinfectants _____, or more often if the solution becomes _____.

37. Porous means _____.

38. List the steps required to disinfect implements.

a. _____.

b. Rinse with water and pat dry.

c. _____.

d. Mix disinfectant according to _____, always adding

_____.

e. _____.

f.  Rinse thoroughly with water and pat dry.

g. _____.

39.  When trying to decide whether to disinfect or dispose of a soiled implement, remember, when in doubt,

_____.

40.  What disinfectant steps should you take before and after each client?

a. _____

b. _____

41.  How do you disinfect a whirlpool pedicure foot spa after each client?

a.  Drain and remove all _____ and _____.

b.  Clean surfaces of the foot spa with _____, and rinse with _____.

c.  Disinfect with an _____, according to _____.

d.  Rinse and wipe dry with a _____.

42.  At the end of each day, what should you do to ensure that your whirlpool foot spa is clean and safe

for use?

a.  Remove and clean the _____ and all _____ trapped behind the _____.

b.  Fill the basin with _____ and _____.

c.  Flush the spa system for _____ then _____ and _____.

d.  Fill with _____ and _____ and circulate through the

basin for _____, then drain and rinse.

e.  Allow the unit to dry _____.

f.  Record the _____ and _____ of the cleaning and disinfecting in the

_____, if required by your state regulatory agency.

43.  What should you do every week to ensure that your whirlpool foot spa remains clean and safe for clients?

a.  Follow the _____ cleaning procedure.

b.  Fill the foot spa tub with water and _____ of _____ bleach solution, based on a

5-gallon tub.

c.  _____ the solution through the foot spa system for _____.

d.  Leave the solution at least _____ hours, or _____.

e.  _____ and _____ the system.

44.  What steps should you take to safely handle a blood spill during a service?

a.  Stop the service and clean the injured area.

b. _____.

c. _____.

d. _____.

e. Clean workstation as necessary.

f. _____

Use a red or orange _____, or a _____.

45. Is it all right to re-use disposable supplies like files, as long as they are still in good shape? _____

_____

_____

46. Before and after _____, hands should be _____.

47. Describe Universal Precautions. _____

_____

_____

## MATCHING REVIEW

*Insert the correct word or term at the left of each definition or description.*

| | | |
|---|---|---|
| sanitizing | asymptomatic | bacteria |
| cocci | diplococci | disinfectant |
| disinfection | fungi | mitosis |
| pathogenic | spirilla | Universal Precautions |
| streptococci | virus | |

48. _____ Centers for Disease Control and Prevention publication

49. _____ first step in the decontamination process

50. _____ infectious submicroscopic organism

51. _____ cell division

52. _____ corkscrew-shaped bacteria

53. _____ disease causing

54. _____ second-highest level of decontamination

55. _____ spherical bacteria

56. _____ used to destroy most bacteria and some viruses

57. _____ microscopic parasites

58. _____ bacteria that cause infections such as blood poisoning

59. _____ most of these one-celled microorganisms are harmless; some are harmful

60. _____ although still contagious, most clients with hepatitis B or other bloodborne diseases show no symptoms of the disease

61. _____ round-shaped bacteria

# General Anatomy and Physiology

## INTRODUCTION

1.  If you are planning on only caring for clients' hands and feet, why is it important to study anatomy?

    _____

    _____

2.  Define anatomy. _____

3.  What is physiology? _____

4.  What is histology? _____

## CELLS

5.  What are cells? Why are they so important? _____

    _____

6.  The human body is made up of _____ of cells that vary widely in _____, _____,

    and _____.

7.  _____ is the fluid content of all living _____. It contains food elements and

    other components, such as _____, _____,

    _____, _____, and _____.

8.  What part of the cell plays an important part in cell reproduction? Where is it located? _____

    _____

9.  What is the name of the watery fluid that surrounds the nucleus? _____

10. What is the function of the cell membrane? _____

    _____

11. When cells reach a certain size they _____ into _____ called _____

    cells. This process is called _____.

12. In order for cells to reproduce, they must:

    a.  Have an adequate supply of _____, _____, and _____

    b.  Have a particular range of _____

    c.  Have the ability to eliminate _____

13. Give two examples of unfavorable conditions that cause cells to become impaired or die:

    _____ and _____.

14. The chemical process that nourishes cells and allows them to carry out their functions is called

    _____.

15. Metabolism has two distinct functions called _____ and _____. Describe these two

    functions.

    a. _____ builds large _____ from _____ ones.

    b. _____ breaks down _____ within the cells into _____.

16. Fill in the blanks with the part of the cell or the cell process that is described or defined. Note: The same

    term may be used more than once.

    a. _____ Basic unit of all living things

    b. _____ Identical cells as a result of mitosis

    c. _____ Allows certain substances to permeate through its walls

    d. _____ Nourishes and enables cells to carry out their duties

    e. _____ There are trillions of them in the human body

    f. _____ Releases stored energy

    g. _____ Found at the center of the cell

    h. _____ Prepares for growth by storing water, food, and oxygen.

    i. _____ Cell division in plants, animals, and bacteria

    j. _____ Constructive metabolism

    k. _____ Without these, life would not exist

    l. _____ The sum of all chemical processes in living cells

    m. _____ Used for growth, reproduction, and self-repair

    n. _____ Dense active protoplasm

    o. _____ Cause cells to become impaired or die

    p. _____ A process describing cell division

## TISSUES

17. Define tissue. _____

18. How many types of tissues are there in the human body? _____ What are their names?

    a. _____

    b. _____

    c. _____

    d. _____

    e. _____

19. What is the function of connective tissue? _____

20. Ligaments, tendons, fascia, and fat are called what? _____

21. The protective covering on the surfaces of the body is called _____. Give four examples of this special covering.

    a. _____

    b. _____

    c. Lining of the _____, _____, and _____ organs

    d. _____

22. Blood and lymph are called _____. They carry _____, _____, and _____ throughout the body.

23. Tissue that contracts and moves the various parts of the body is called _____.

24. _____ transmits messages to and from the _____. It is composed of special cells known as _____.

25. _____ are the basic working units of the nervous system.

## ORGANS

26. What are organs? _____

27. List the function of the following eight major organs.

    a. Brain _____

    b. Eyes _____

    c. Heart _____

    d. Kidneys _____

    e. Lungs _____

    f. Liver _____

    g. Skin _____

    h. Stomach and intestines _____

## BODY SYSTEMS

28. What is meant by body systems? _____

29. Identify the ten major systems of the human body based on the descriptions below.

    a. _____ Pertaining to the heart, blood vessels, and the circulation of blood

    b. _____ Changes food into nutrients and wastes

    c. _____ Ductless glands that regulate bodily functions via hormones secreted into the bloodstream

    d. _____ Purifies the body by eliminating waste matter

    e. _____ Protective covering that also helps regulate body temperature

f. _____ System that allows the body to move internally and externally

g. _____ Controls and coordinates all other systems

h. _____ Specific organs that regulate all sexual functioning

i. _____ Enables breathing, supplies the body with oxygen, and eliminates carbon dioxide as a waste product

j. _____ The physical foundation of the body

30. **Matching.** *Match the terms on the left with descriptions on the right. Note: The same word or term may have more than one answer.*

_____ 1. tissue

_____ 2. adipose tissue

_____ 3. systems

_____ 4. connective tissue

_____ 5. liquid tissue

_____ 6. epithelial tissue

_____ 7. organs

_____ 8. nerve tissue

_____ 9. muscular tissue

A. bone, cartilage, ligament, and tendons

B. five major types in the human body

C. allows the body to contract and move

D. groups of organs that work together

E. moves food and waste through the body

F. skin and mucous membranes

G. controls and coordinates all bodily functions

H. lining of the heart, digestive, and respiratory organs

I. collection of similar cells

J. fat

K. groups of tissues that perform a specific function

31. **Matching.** *Match the terms on the left with descriptions on the right.*

_____ 1. respiratory

_____ 2. digestive

_____ 3. muscular

_____ 4. excretory

_____ 5. nervous

_____ 6. integumentary

_____ 7. circulatory

_____ 8. reproductive

_____ 9. skeletal

_____ 10. endocrine

A. ductless glands that regulate bodily functions

B. lungs and air passages

C. brain, spinal cord and nerves

D. mouth, esophagus, stomach, liver, among others

E. made up of muscles

F. skin, hair and nails

G. eliminates waste via kidneys, liver, among others

H. pertaining to the heart and blood vessels

I. specific organs that regulate all sexual functioning

J. bones and cartilages

## THE SKELETAL SYSTEM

32. What is the skeletal system? _____

33. Define osteology. _____

34. How many bones make up the skeletal system? _____

35. Bone is the hardest tissue in the body except for what? _____

36. What are bones made of? _____

37. What are the two major minerals found in bones? _____

38. List the six major functions of the skeletal system.

    a.   Gives _____ and _____ to the body

    b.   Protects _____ and _____

    c.   Serves as _____ for muscles

    d.   Acts as _____ to produce _____

    e.   Helps produce both _____ and _____ blood cells

    f.   Stores most of the body's _____

39. A connection between two or more bones is called a _____.

40. Name the two types of joints and cite at least two examples of each.

    a.   _____

    b.   _____

41. Name and describe the bones of the arms.

    a.   _____

    b.   _____

    c.   _____

42. Name and describe the bones of the hand.

    a.   _____

    b.   _____

    c.   _____

43. **Matching.** *Match the terms on the left with descriptions on the right.*

| | | |
|---|---|---|
| _____ 1. humerus | A. | lower arm bone, same side as thumb |
| _____ 2. ulna | B. | bones of the palm of the hand |
| _____ 3. radius | C. | flexible joint made up of eight small bones |
| _____ 4. carpus | D. | three bones in each finger and each toe |
| _____ 5. metacarpus | E. | largest bone of the arm |
| _____ 6. phalanges | F. | inner bone of the forearm, attached to the wrist |

44. **Matching.** *Match the terms on the left with the descriptions on the right.*

| | | |
|---|---|---|
| _____ 1. tibia | A. | bones that compose the toes |
| _____ 2. femur | B. | long and slender bones |
| _____ 3. tarsal | C. | heavy, long bone that forms the leg above the knee |
| _____ 4. fibula | D. | smaller of two bones that forms the leg below the knee |

_____ 5. phalanges          E.  there are seven of these bones in the foot

_____ 6. patella            F.  ankle bone

_____ 7. talus              G.  larger of two bones that forms the leg below the knee

_____ 8. metatarsal         H.  forms the kneecap joint

## THE MUSCULAR SYSTEM

45.  What is the muscular system? _____

46.  What are muscles made of? How do they work? _____

_____

47.  Define myology. _____

48.  Approximately how many muscles are in the human body? _____

49.  Name and define the three types of muscular tissue.

　　 a.  _____

　　 b.  _____

　　 c.  _____

50.  Name and describe the three parts of a muscle.

　　 a.  _____

　　 b.  _____

　　 c.  _____

51.  List seven ways that muscles can be stimulated.

　　 a.  _____ using _____ or electric _____

　　 b.  _____ or _____ electric current

　　 c.  _____ or _____ light

　　 d.  _____ such as heating _____

　　 e.  _____ such as _____ or warm _____

　　 f.  _____ through the nervous system

　　 g.  _____, including certain _____ or salts

52.  What are the names of the muscles that attach the arms to the body? Which movements do they control?

　　 a.  _____

　　 b.  _____

　　 c.  _____

　　 d.  _____

_____

53. The shoulders and upper arms have three principal muscles. What are they? What do they do?

   a. _____

   b. _____

   c. _____

54. The forearm has a series of muscles. What are they? What do they do?

   a. _____

   b. _____

   c. _____

   d. _____

55. The hand is made up of many small muscles that overlap from joint to joint. Why?

   _____

56. There are two important muscles of the hand. What are they? What do they do?

   a. _____

   b. _____

57. **True and False.** *Insert T or F in the space at the left.*

_____ 1. Muscle accounts for approximately 40% of the body's weight.

_____ 2. Pectoralis major and pectoralis minor are chest muscles.

_____ 3. Biceps lift the forearm and flex the elbow.

_____ 4. Extensors cause the wrist, hand, and fingers to contract.

_____ 5. Muscles can stretch and contract.

_____ 6. The supinator turns the palm upward.

_____ 7. Nonstriated muscles are attached to bone.

_____ 8. Triceps are responsible for extending the elbow.

_____ 9. Massage normally applies pressure from the insertion point to the origin.

_____ 10. The involuntary heart muscle is called the cardiac muscle.

_____ 11. Abductors and adductors are arm muscles.

_____ 12. Pronators turn the hand downward so that the palm faces up.

_____ 13. Muscular tissue cannot be stimulated by massage.

_____ 14. A muscle has four parts.

_____ 15. Adductors draw the fingers together.

_____ 16. Dry heat, moist heat, and nerve impulses can stimulate muscular tissue.

_____ 17. Electrical current cannot penetrate into muscle tissue.

_____ 18. Nonstriated muscles function voluntarily.

_____ 19. Striated muscles help maintain posture.

58. **Matching.** *Match the terms on the left with the descriptions on the right.*

_____ 1. extensor digitorum longis     A. bends the foot upward and inward

_____ 2. peroneus brevis     B. inverts the foot and turns it outward

_____ 3. tibialis anterior     C. bends the foot up and extends the toes

_____ 4. gastrocnemius     D. bends the foot down

_____ 5. peroneus longus     E. pulls the foot down

_____ 6. soleus     F. bends the foot down and out

## THE NERVOUS SYSTEM

59. What is the nervous system? _____

_____

60. There are over _____ nerve cells, known as _____, in the human body.

61. The nervous system is divided into three parts. What are they? What do they do?

a. _____

_____

b. _____

_____

c. _____

_____

62. What is the largest and most complex nerve tissue in the body? _____

63. Where is the brain anatomically located? What does it control? _____

_____

64. The spinal cord belongs to which nervous system? Where is it located? _____

_____

65. The primary structural unit of a nerve cell is called a(n) _____. Each one of these has

_____, _____, and the _____.

66. What is a nerve? _____

_____

67. Name the two types of nerves and what they do.

a. _____

_____

b. _____

_____

68. Define reflex. _____

69. Name the four principal nerves that supply the superficial parts of the arm and and the back.

a. _____

b. _____

c. _____

d. _____

70. **True and False.** *Insert T or F in the space at the left.*

_____ 1. Sensory nerves called receptors are located close to the surface of the skin.

_____ 2. The principal components of the nervous system are the brain, spinal cord, and liver.

_____ 3. Every square centimeter of the human body is supplied with fine fibers known as nerves.

_____ 4. An understanding of how nerves work will help you perform services in a more proficient manner.

_____ 5. The brain weighs more than 5 pounds.

_____ 6. Motor nerves produce movement.

_____ 7. Median nerves supply the arm and hand.

_____ 8. Dendrites receive impulses from other neurons.

_____ 9. Axons send impulses to other nerve cells.

_____ 10. The central nervous system controls the involuntary muscles.

_____ 11. The central nervous system controls consciousness and many mental activities.

_____ 12. Digital nerves supply the fingers.

71. **Matching.** *Match the terms on the left with the descriptions on the right.*

_____ 1. tibial nerve      A. supplies impulses to the skin on top of the foot

_____ 2. saphenous nerve      B. divides into two branches

_____ 3. dorsal nerve      C. supplies impulses to muscles and skin of the leg

_____ 4. sural nerve      D. supplies impulses to skin of inner side of the leg and foot

_____ 5. common peroneal nerve      E. supplies impulses adjacent to sides of the first and second toes

_____ 6. superficial peroneal nerve      F. supplies impulses to skin on outer side and back of foot and leg

_____ 7. deep peroneal nerve      G. supplies impulses to the knee, calf, sole, and heel

# THE CIRCULATORY SYSTEM

72. The circulatory system is also referred to as the _____ or _____.

73. What does the circulatory system do? _____

_____

74. The circulatory system is made up of two parts. What are these parts and what do they do?

a. _____

_____

b. _____

_____

## The Heart

75. The heart is a _____ organ that is often referred to as the body's _____. It is surrounded by a membrane called the _____.

76. The heart beats between _____ and _____ times per minute when _____.

77. The heart is made up of four _____ and four _____.

78. The upper chambers, called the _____ and _____, have _____ walls. The lower chambers, called the _____ and the _____, have _____ walls.

79. The _____ are located between the _____. They keep the blood flowing _____.

80. Name the two systems that are responsible for circulating blood throughout the body. What does each system do?

a. _____

b. _____

## Blood Vessels

81. What are blood vessels? _____

82. There are three types of blood vessels. Name them and describe their functions.

a. _____

_____

b. _____

_____

c. _____

_____

## The Blood

83. What is blood? Blood is a nutritive fluid containing _____, _____, _____, _____, and _____. It is comprised of 80%- _____.

84. There are approximately _____ to _____ pints of blood in the human body.

85. How can you tell whether blood is oxygen rich or oxygen poor? _____

_____

86. What do red blood cells do? _____

87. What is the primary function of white blood cells? _____

88. What is the primary function of platelets? _____

89. Plasma is the _____ part of the _____. It carries _____ and other important sub-

stances to the _____, and takes away _____ from the _____.

90. Describe the five primary functions of blood.

    a. _____

    b. _____

    c. _____

    d. _____

    e. _____

91. Which two arteries provide the main blood supply of the arms and hands?

    a. _____

    b. _____

92. Describe the lymph vascular system. _____

93. List the primary functions of the lymph vascular system.

    a. Defends against invading _____ and _____

    b. Removes _____ from the _____

    c. Provides a suitable _____ environment for the _____

    d. Carries _____ from the _____ to the _____

94. **Matching.** *Match the terms on the left with descriptions on the right.*

    _____ 1. vein                          A. destroys disease-causing microorganisms

    _____ 2. artery                        B. red and white cells, platelets, plasma, etc.

    _____ 3. blood                         C. responsible for blood clotting

    _____ 4. white blood cells             D. lines the heart

    _____ 5. plasma                        E. fluid part of the blood

    _____ 6. hemoglobin                    F. aorta

    _____ 7. circulatory system            G. allows the blood to flow in only one direction

    _____ 8. ulnar artery, radial artery   H. the body's pump

    _____ 9. pulmonary circulation         I. sends blood from the heart to the lungs

    _____ 10. heart                        J. blood supply to the arm and hand

    _____ 11. pericardium                  K. moves waste products back toward the heart

_____ 12. heart valves

_____ 13. lymphatic system

_____ 14. platelets

L.   complex iron protein that binds to oxygen

M.   lymph, lymphatics, lymph nodes

N.   heart, arteries, veins and capillaries

## THE ENDOCRINE SYSTEM

95.   Define endocrine glands. _____

_____

96.   Sweat and oil glands belong to this system. True or False? _____

## THE DIGESTIVE SYSTEM

97.   What is the function of the digestive system? _____

_____

98.   How is food digested? _____

99.   How long does it generally take for the digestive system to completely process food? _____

## THE EXCRETORY SYSTEM

100.   What is the primary function of the excretory system? _____

101.   Explain the functions of the organs included in the excretory system.

a.   Kidneys _____ .

b.   Skin _____ .

c.   Large intestine _____ .

d.   Lungs _____ .

e.   Liver _____ .

## THE RESPIRATORY SYSTEM

102.   The respiratory system involves the _____ and _____. List and describe its two phases.

a.   _____

b.   _____

103.   You can survive _____ or longer without food, _____ without water, but only a

_____ without oxygen.

104.   The term "respiration" means _____ .

105.   The _____ helps control breathing.

## THE INTEGUMENTARY SYSTEM

106.   What makes up the integumentary system? _____

_____

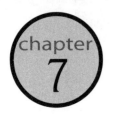

# Skin Structure and Growth

## INTRODUCTION

1. What is the largest organ of the body? _____

2. Describe the four characteristics of healthy skin.

   a. _____

   b. _____

   c. _____

   d. _____

## ANATOMY OF THE SKIN

3. Label the different parts of the skin.

   1. _____

   2. _____

   3. _____

   4. _____

   5. _____

   6. _____

   7. _____

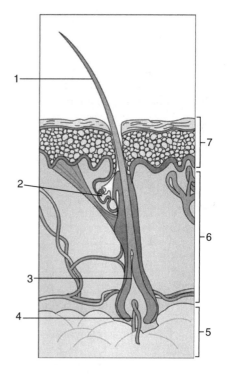

4. Label the layers and sub-layers of the skin.

   a. _____

   _____

   _____

   b. _____

   c. _____

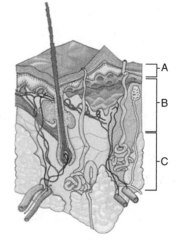

5. **Identification.** *Using the letters **E, D**, or **H** (defined below), match the descriptions to the correct layer of skin.*

   **Key:**                          **Characteristics:**

   **E** = epidermis                 _____ 1. Contains two separate layers

   **D** = dermis                    _____ 2. Blood vessels, nerves, sweat and oil glands are found in
                                               this layer

   **S** = Subcutaneous              _____ 3. Cuticle layer

                                     _____ 4. Has four layers, each of which is called a stratum

                                     _____ 5. Deep layer of the skin

                                     _____ 6. Papillary, reticular

                                     _____ 7. Contains nerve endings but no blood vessels

                                     _____ 8. Adipose tissue is found here

                                     _____ 9. Outer layer of the skin

                                     _____ 10. Also called true skin, corium, or cutis

                                     _____ 11. Keratinized cells are found here

6. What are the three primary purposes of subcutaneous tissue?

   a. _____

   b. _____

   c. _____

### How the Skin Is Nourished

7. _____ and _____ are carried through the bloodstream to the skin. These _____

   include molecules of _____, _____, and _____ derived from food.

8. Define lymph. _____

   _____

9. _____ bathes the _____, removes _____ and _____, and provides

   _____ properties for the skin.

### Nerves of the Skin

10. Match the different types of nerve fibers with their functions.

   _____ 1. motor          A. react to heat, cold, touch, pressure and pain

   _____ 2. sensory        B. regulate the flow of sebum and perspiration

   _____ 3. secretory      C. distributed to the arrector pili muscles

### Sense of Touch

11. Nerve endings that produce the sense of touch are situated in what layer of the skin?

   _____

12. What different sensations do these nerve endings allow us to feel? _____

13. Which area of the hand has the largest number of nerve endings? _____

14. Motor nerve fibers are distributed to the _____ attached to the hair follicles, which can cause goose bumps when a person is frightened or cold.

## Skin Color

15. The pigment-causing substance in the skin is called _____. It is found in the _____ of the _____.

16. There are two types of this pigment that produce different depths of skin color. What are they?

    a. _____ Red to yellow in color, people with light-complexioned skin mostly produce this type of pigment.

    b. _____ Brown to black in color, people with dark-complexioned skin mostly produce this type of pigment.

17. Melanin helps to protect skin cells against harmful UV rays. True or false? _____

## Strength and Flexibility of the Skin

18. Define collagen and elastin. _____ These two structures make up _____ of the dermis.

19. What are their functions?

    a. Collagen gives the skin _____.

    b. Elastin allows the skin to _____.

20. When collagen fibers are healthy, they allow the skin to _____ and _____.

21. What are some of the reasons that collagen loses its resiliency, leading to wrinkles and flaccid or sagging skin?

    a. _____

    b. _____

    c. _____

## Glands of the Skin

22. The following two types of duct glands extract materials from the blood to form new substances. What do they produce?

    a. Sudoriferous or sweat glands. _____

    b. Sebaceous or oil glands. _____

23. **Identification.** *Using the letters **SU** and **SE** (defined below), match the correct characteristics with the correct gland.*

**Key:**

**SU**=sudoriferous gland

**SE**=sebaceous gland

**Characteristics:**

_____ 1. eliminates one to two pints of liquid daily

_____ 2. not found on the palms or soles

_____ 3. regulates body temperature

_____ 4. lubricates skin and softens hair

_____ 5. palms, soles, forehead, and armpits have the greatest number of them

_____ 6. a blackhead may form

_____ 7. has a coiled base or secretory coil

_____ 8. secretes sebum

_____ 9. opens into the hair follicle

_____ 10. eliminates waste

## FUNCTIONS OF THE SKIN

24. Name and explain the principal functions of the skin.

   a. _____

   b. _____

   c. _____

   d. _____

   e. _____

   f. _____

## AGING OF THE SKIN

25. What happens to collagen and elastin fibers as we age? _____

26. What effect does the prolonged exposure of UV rays have on the skin's melanin? _____

_____

27. What percentage does heredity generally contribute to visible skin aging? _____

28. What is the primary factor in skin aging? _____

29. What precautions should you share with your clients to help prevent sun damage and premature aging?

   a. Wear a _____, _____ sunscreen.

   b. Avoid _____ between 10:00 AM and 3:00 PM, the hours when _____ is highest.

   c. Apply sunscreen approximately _____ before going out in the sun.

   d. Always reapply sunscreen after _____.

e. Always check the _____ on the bottle to ensure that it has not _____.

f. Children _____ should not be exposed to the _____.

g. Have a regular _____ check-up by a _____ to ensure that no

   _____ or _____ lesions are present.

h. Moles that have undergone a change in _____, _____, or _____, pigmented

   spots with _____ borders, or skin that unexpectedly _____ or

   _____ should be immediately checked by a dermatologist.

i. In between doctor's appointments, do a _____ at home.

### Skin Aging and the Environment

30. What types of environmental issues, besides sun exposure, can lead to premature aging of the skin?

   _____

31. Do these pollutants only affect the surface of the skin? Please explain. _____

   _____

32. What is the best defense against pollutants? _____

33. Skin aging is also caused by poor lifestyle choices. Name four.

   a. _____

   b. _____

   c. _____

   d. _____

## SKIN DISORDERS

34. Why do nail technicians need to learn about skin disorders? _____

   _____

   _____

35. The only person qualified to diagnose a disorder/disease is a _____.

### Lesions of the Skin

36. What are lesions? _____

37. There are three types of lesions: _____, _____, and _____. Nail technicians

   should only be concerned about _____ and _____ lesions.

38. Once you become familiar with various lesions, you will be able to distinguish between conditions that

   _____ or _____ be treated in a salon.

39. **Matching.** *Match the primary lesions at the left to the descriptions on the right.*

   _____ 1. tubercle        A. large blister containing watery fluid

   _____ 2. macule          B. closed, fluid-filled mass below the surface of the skin

38

_____ 3. cyst     C. pimple; small skin swelling that sometimes contains pus

_____ 4. papule     D. flat, discolored spot such as a freckle; flat rash

_____ 5. tumor     E. small blister or sac containing clear fluid

_____ 6. vesicle     F. inflamed, pus-filled pimple

_____ 7. wheal     G. abnormal mass caused by excessive multiplication of cells

_____ 8. bulla     H. itchy, swollen lesion that lasts only a few hours

_____ 9. pustule     I. round, solid lump that can be above or below the skin; larger than a papule

40. **Matching.** Secondary lesions appear in the later stages of diseases or disorders. *Match the secondary lesions at the left to the descriptions at the right.*

_____ 1. crust     A. chapped hands

_____ 2. excoriation     B. an open lesion on the skin

_____ 3. fissure     C. scratch

_____ 4. scale     D. a mark on the skin formed after an injury

_____ 5. scar or cicatrix     E. epidermal flakes, dry or oily, such as dandruff

_____ 6. ulcer     F. dead cells that form over wounds while healing

### *Disorders of the Sudoriferous (Sweat) Glands*

41. **Matching.** *Match the conditions on the left with the proper description or definition on the right.*

_____ 1. anhidrosis     A. sudden eruption of small red vesicles that burn and itch; commonly called prickly heat

_____ 2. bromhidrosis     B. a disorder characterized by the inability to sweat

_____ 3. miliaria ruba     C. offensive body odor, especially from armpits and feet

## INFLAMMATIONS OF THE SKIN

42. Dermatitis is an _____ of the skin such as _____ or _____.

43. _____ is an inflammatory, painful itching disease of the skin, presenting many forms of dry or moist lesions.

44. Psoriasis is a non-contagious condition characterized by _____ patches covered with _____ scales. Psoriasis is typically found on the _____, _____, _____, _____, and _____.

## SKIN CONDITIONS

45. There are many kinds of dermatitis, but only one is important to nail technicians: _____.

46. Name two types of contact dermatitis:

    a. _____.

    b. _____.

47. Allergic reactions are caused by _____ and _____ skin contact. List the likely

    places for allergies to occur on the nail technician:

    a. _____

    b. _____

    c. _____

48. Define sensitization. _____

49. The risk of sensitization does not increase with each service. True or False _____

50. In general, it takes from _____ to _____ months of repeated exposure before sensitive

    clients show symptoms.

51. Prolonged, repeated or long term exposures can cause anyone to become sensitive, this is usually caused

    by _____.

    a. Between the thumb and index finger: _____

    b. Back of forearm: _____

    c. Palms: _____

    d. Face: _____

52. Touching clients' skin with any _____ or _____ during nail services is the most common

    reason for client _____. List the causes of such contact.

    a. Not leaving a _____ free margin between the product and skin

    b. Overly _____ product consistency

    c. Inadequate curing of UV gel due to _____

    d. Incomplete curing of UV gel by _____

    e. Applying the product _____

    f. Using _____ brushes

53. To ensure that your UV bulbs are adequately curing the product:

    a. Replace them at least _____ per year.

    b. Use the lamp that is designed _____.

    c. _____ the surfaces of the bulbs _____.

54. Give examples of irritants that can cause irritant contact dermatitis. _____

55. Avoiding _____ and _____ contact with an irritating substance, the skin will

    _____. Prolonged exposure, though, can lead to _____.

56. Because nail enhancement products are not designed for _____, take extreme care to keep

    _____, _____ and _____ clean and free from product dusts and residues.

## Pigment-Related Skin Conditions

57. **Matching.** *Match the following skin conditions to the appropriate descriptions or definitions on the right.*

_____ 1.  albinism

_____ 2.  lentigines

_____ 3.  leukoderma

_____ 4.  nevus

_____ 5.  stain

_____ 6.  tan

_____ 7.  vitiligo

A.  caused by a burn or congenital disease

B.  absence of melanin of the body; pink eyes

C.  darkening of skin due to exposure to UV rays

D.  birthmark; malformation due to dilated capillaries

E.  milky-white spots

F.  permanent brown or wine-colored skin discoloration

G.  freckles

## Hypertrophies of the Skin

58.  What is a hypertrophy of the skin? _____

59.  Are all hypertrophies benign? _____

60.  What is a keratoma? _____

61.  Describe a mole. _____

62.  When does a mole require medical attention? _____

63.  What is a skin tag? _____

64.  Define verruca. _____. What causes a verruca to appear? _____

65.  Verrucas are contagious. True or false. _____

## Skin Cancer

66.  Skin cancer is primarily caused by _____.

67.  There are three distinct forms of skin cancer. List them from the least to the most serious. Provide a general description of each.

a.  _____

b.  _____

c.  _____

68.  _____ is called a "city person's cancer" because it often appears on parts of the

body that do not regularly receive _____.

## MAINTAINING SKIN HEALTH

69.  _____ are essential to maintaining _____.

70.  Vitamins _____, _____, _____, and _____ have been proven to positively impact the health of the skin.

71.  Although experts agree that taking vitamins _____ is still the best way to support the health of

the skin, some _____ applications of vitamins have also been found useful in nourishing the skin.

72. The best source of vitamin D is limited amounts of _____.

73. Vitamin C speeds up the body's _____.

74. _____ and _____ supplements help meet the body's daily _____ needs.

### Water and the Skin

75. _____ to _____ percent of the body's weight is comprised of _____.

76. The health of the cell is sustained by drinking _____.

77. Water aids in the _____ of toxins and waste, helps regulate the body's _____ and aids in _____.

78. **True or false.** *Insert T or F to the left of each statement below.*

_____ 1. Metabolism can be slowed by as much as 3%- with even mild dehydration.

_____ 2. Daytime fatigue is not affected by water content.

_____ 3. Short-term memory is related to hormones, not water.

_____ 4. Feelings of hunger can be lessened by drinking a glass of water.

_____ 5. Drinking lots of water can help stop hunger pangs for many dieters.

chapter

8

Date _____

Rating _____

Text Pages 138–143

# Nail Structure and Growth

## INTRODUCTION

1. The natural nail is the _____

2. What are nails made out of? _____

3. Describe what a healthy nail should look like. _____

   _____

4. What is the water content of a healthy nail? _____

5. What does an adequate amount of water do for the nail? _____

6. What does an inadequate amount of water cause? _____

7. What steps can a nail technician take to lower water loss in the nails? _____

   _____

## NAIL ANATOMY

8. Label the parts of the nail.

   1. _____

   2. _____

   3. _____

   4. _____

   5. _____

   6. _____

9. **Matching.** *Match the nail parts on the left with descriptions on the right.*

_____ 1. nail plate

_____ 2. nail fold

_____ 3. lunula

_____ 4. bed epithelium

_____ 5. keratin

_____ 6. specialized ligaments

_____ 7. free edge

A. folds of skin that surround the nail plate

B. dead colorless tissue attached to the nail plate

C. portion of living skin on which the nail plate sits

D. creates a seal to prevent microorganisms from invading and infecting the nail bed

E. attaches the nail to the nail plate

F. most visible and functional part of the nail

G. bottom skin of each toe

_____ 8. grooves      H. produces the nail plate

_____ 9. hyponychium      I. slits or furrows on which the nail moves

_____ 10. matrix bed      J. the living skin at the base of the nail plate

_____ 11. eponychium      K. bottom skin of each finger

_____ 12. nail bed      L. extends over the tip of the finger or toe

_____ 13. cuticle      M. where the natural nail is formed

N. nails are made of this protein

O. visible part of the matrix, extending from underneath the living skin

P. attaches the nail bed and matrix bed to the underlying bone

10. Poor nail growth is caused by what factors?

a. _____

b. _____

c. _____

11. How is the nail plate formed? _____

12. A nail plate consists of about _____ layers of _____ .

13. The main job of the cuticle is to: (*Circle the correct answer.*)

a. Prevent infection and injury

b. Hold the nail in place

c. Help shape the nail

14. Name the parts of the natural nail unit.

a. _____

b. _____

c. _____

d. _____

e. _____

## NAIL GROWTH

15. What affects nail growth?

a. _____

b. _____

c. _____

16. What determines the thickness, width, and curvature of the nail plate? _____

_____

17. What does a longer matrix produce? _____

18. What does a highly curved matrix produce? _____

19. Normal adults can expect their nails to grow about _____ or _____ per month.

20. Nails grow faster in the summer than they do in the winter. True or false? _____

21. What nail grows the fastest? _____

22. What nail grows the slowest? _____

23. Which grow fastest overall: toenails or fingernails? _____

24. After losing a toenail, how long does it take for a new nail to completely take its place? _____

25. How long does ordinary replacement of the natural nail take? _____

Date _____

Rating _____

Text Pages 144–155

# Nail Diseases and Disorders

## INTRODUCTION

1. What is a nail disorder? _____

2. To provide a safe environment for clients, nail technicians must _____

   _____

3. If the disorder is not a medical condition, you may be able to _____ certain nail plate conditions.

4. List and describe four symptoms that would prohibit nail services.

   a. _____

   b. _____

   c. _____

   d. _____

5. **Matching.** *Match the nail disorders on the left with the descriptions on the right.*

   _____ 1. bruised nails           A. noticeably thin, more flexible than normal

   _____ 2. ridges                  B. horizontal depressions caused by illness or trauma

   _____ 3. eggshell nails          C. white spots not related to health

   _____ 4. beau lines              D. deep or sharp curvature at the free edge

   _____ 5. hangnail or agnail      E. abnormal rough nail plate

   _____ 6. leukonychia spots       F. skin is stretched by the nail plate

   _____ 7. melanonychia            G. folded nail

   _____ 8. onychophagy             H. split cuticle

   _____ 9. onychorrhexis           I. nails bitten to the point of deformity

   _____ 10. plicatured nail        J. black bands underneath the nail plate

   _____ 11. nail pterygium         K. furrows running the length or width of the nail

   _____ 12. trumpet or pincer nail  L. clot forms underneath the nail plate

   _____ 13. nail psoriasis         M. maybe a stain or an internal problem

   _____ 14. discolored nails       N. nail pitting

   _____ 15. onychocryptosis        O. ingrown nails

6. What symptoms indicate that a client should seek medical attention for a hangnail? _____

_____

7. When nail bruising occurs, the _____ absorbs the _____ and the resulting stain _____ with the nail.

8. Internal disease, hereditary factors, medication, and improper diet can also result in _____.

9. What is an ingrown nail or _____? What can you do to alleviate this condition?

_____

_____

10. When treating eggshell nails, you should always use the _____ side of an abrasive board. This means _____ grit or less.

11. Pneumonia, adverse drug reactions, surgery, heart failure, massive injury, and high fevers can result in _____.

12. _____ are visible depressions resulting from major illness or injury that will usually disappear once nail plate thickness returns to normal.

13. When the living skin splits around the nail, it is called a _____ or _____.

14. Hangnails can be corrected with proper _____.

15. Leukonychia are _____ that _____ indicate disease. They are caused by a _____.

16. A localized area of increased pigment cells within the matrix bed is usually responsible for _____. It is common in _____ clients.

17. Severe cases of nail biting can result in _____, a condition where the skin surrounding the _____ is _____.

18. Split or brittle nails with a series of lengthwise ridges is called _____. Name six reasons for this disorder.

    a. _____

    b. _____

    c. _____

    d. _____

    e. _____

    f. _____

19. The above condition can be corrected by _____ the use of harsh _____, _____, _____, or improper filing of the nail plate. Using a high-quality, penetrating _____ can be beneficial.

20. Abnormal damage to the eponychium or hyponychium is called _____.

21. Never treat _____ by pushing back the _____ of skin.

22. A type of highly curved nail plate often caused by injury to the matrix is called _____. It figuratively means _____ nail.

## NAIL FUNGUS

23. What are fungi? _____

24. Fungi are more easily spread on the _____ than on the hands. They are easily transmitted through _____.

25. Clients with fungus should be _____ for treatment.

26. Referring to the discoloration between the _____ and an _____ as a mold is _____. It is actually a _____ infection.

27. Bacterial infections can thrive on nails _____ than _____ infections.

28. These infections are a result of moisture trapped between the nail and the enhancement. True or false? _____

29. A _____ spot on the nail indicates an early _____ infection.

30. A _____ spot indicates a more advanced _____ infection.

31. _____ and _____ infections can be avoided when you perform proper _____ and _____ procedures.

## NAIL DISEASES

32. When inflammation is evident around the matrix, the condition is referred to as _____. It can be caused by improperly _____ and _____ nail implements.

33. What types of careers or jobs are more likely to cause nail infections? _____

_____

34. Because they spend a lot of time in a warm, moist environment, toenails are most susceptible to _____ infections.

35. What causes the nail to lift away from the bed without shedding? What is this condition called?

_____

_____

36. What could you be doing during a nail service to cause the above condition? _____ or _____.

37. If there is no indication of an infection or breaks in the skin, clients with _____ can receive gentle _____ and _____ services.

38. Clients who have skin psoriasis often have _____. Characteristics can include:

   a. _____

   b. _____

   c. _____

   d. _____

   e. _____

39. A lump of _____ tissue growing up from the nail bed to the nail plate, indicating severe infection, is called _____.

40. Fungal infections of the feet are called _____. They are characterized by:

   a. _____

   b. _____

41. Clients with foot fungus should be advised to:

   a. _____ their feet every day and _____ them completely.

   b. Wear _____ socks.

   c. Change socks _____.

   d. Use an over-the-counter _____.

   e. Avoid wearing the same _____ every day.

42. What is a fungal infection of the natural nail plate called? _____

# Basics of Chemistry

## INTRODUCTION

1. Without _____, most nail services would not be possible.

2. Why is it important to have a basic knowledge of chemistry? _____

3. What is chemistry? _____

   _____

4. What is organic chemistry? _____

5. All living things, whether they are plant or animal, contain _____.

6. What is inorganic chemistry? _____

   _____

7. Any substance that occupies space is called _____.

8. All _____ has physical properties that we can _____, _____, or _____.

9. We can also see some forms of energy such as _____.

10. What is an element? _____

    _____. There are _____ naturally occurring ele-

    ments, each with its own distinctive _____ and _____ properties.

11. A letter symbol is assigned to each element: for example, O is for _____, C for _____, H

    for _____, N for _____, and S for _____.

12. Elements are differentiated by the _____.

13. All matter is composed of _____.

14. When two or more atoms are joined together, they form a _____.

15. When two or more elements are chemically joined together, they form a _____.

16. Matter exists in three forms. Name these forms and describe them.

    a. _____.

    b. _____.

    c. _____.

17. Depending on its temperature, _____ assumes one of these _____. Example: Water turn-

    ing to steam. It does not turn into another _____; it simply changes _____.

## PHYSICAL AND CHEMICAL PROPERTIES OF MATTER

18. Name the two ways that matter can be changed: _____.

19. Changing the _____ of substances does not chemically alter them. An example is ice. When it melts, it physically changes into water, but the chemical makeup remains the same.

20. Two examples of chemical changes are the oxidation of _____ and the polymerization of

    _____.

## PURE SUBSTANCES AND PHYSICAL MIXTURES

21. What is a physical mixture? _____

    _____

22. What is a pure substance? _____

## SOLUTIONS, SUSPENSIONS, AND EMULSIONS

23. Physical mixtures that contain two or more different substances are called _____, _____,

    or _____.

24. A stable mixture of two or more _____ is called a _____.

25. A substance dissolved in a solution is called a _____.

26. A substance that dissolves another substance to form a solution is called a _____.

27. Miscible liquids are _____ soluble.

28. Liquids that can be mixed with each other without separating are called _____ liquids. Example: water and alcohol.

29. Water and oil are examples of _____ liquids because they _____ upon standing.

30. Stable solutions do not _____.

31. Tiny, solid particles finely distributed through a liquid form a _____. A common example of this is oil-and-vinegar salad dressing.

32. When two or more immiscible substances unite with the aid of a binder or emulsifier, it is called an

    _____.

33. Define emulsify. _____

34. Surfactant is a contraction for the term _____.

35. Name and define the two distinct parts of a surfactant.

    a. _____

    b. _____

36. In chemistry, like dissolves like. What does this mean? _____

37. An atom or molecule that carries an electrical charge is called an _____.

38. _____ causes an atom or molecule to split in two, creating a pair of ions with opposite electrical charges.

39. An _____ is an ion with a negative electrical charge.

40. A _____ is an ion with a positive electrical charge.

41. Some molecules naturally ionize into _____ ions and _____ ions in water.

42. Because hydroxide ions are _____, they influence the _____ of water.

43. Only products that contain _____ can have a pH.

44. When the same number of hydrogen ions and hydroxide ions are present, the solution is _____.

45. The pH of any substance is always a balance of both _____ and _____.

46. Pure water is _____ % acid and _____ % alkaline.

47. The pH scale goes from 0 to 14, with 7 being neutral. Below 7, the solution is _____, and above 7 it is _____

48. Hair and skin have an average pH of _____.

49. **Matching.** *Match the terms on the left with the descriptions on the right.*

_____ 1. anion

_____ 2. alkanolamines

_____ 3. exothermic

_____ 4. water-in-oil-emulsion

_____ 5. oxidizing agent

_____ 6. miscible

_____ 7. neutral

_____ 8. hydrogen ion

_____ 9. emulsion

_____ 10. hydroxide ion

_____ 11. neutral

_____ 12. ammonia

_____ 13. cation

_____ 14. chemical change

_____ 15. hydrophilic

_____ 16. volatile organic compounds (VOCs)

_____ 17. immiscible

_____ 18. silicones

A. base

B. equal proportions of acids and alkalis

C. chemical reaction producing heat

D. substance that releases oxygen

E. equal number of hydrogen and hydroxide ions

F. alkaline

G. acidic

H. negatively charged ion

I. positive charged ion

J. colorless gas with a pungent odor

K. substances that neutralize acids

L. compounds containing carbon that evaporate quickly

M. water-resistant lubricants for the skin

N. fatty alcohol

O. water droplets suspended in an oil base

P. water loving

_____ 19. matter

_____ 20. molecule

_____ 21. cetyl alcohol

_____ 22. physical change

_____ 23. lipophilic

_____ 24. solution

_____ 25. alkali

_____ 26. atom

Q.  oil loving

R.  oil droplets suspended in a water base

S.  capable of being mixed into stable solutions

T.  water and oil

U.  change in chemical composition

V.  solid dissolved in a liquid

W.  no chemical reaction is involved

X.  two or more atoms chemically joined together

Y.  anything that occupies space

Z.  basic component of all matter

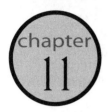

Date _____

Rating _____

Text Pages 174–185

# Nail Product Chemistry Simplified

## INTRODUCTION

1. Knowing how to _____ and _____ common service problems is dependent on your basic understanding of the _____ of your products.

2. Most chemicals are dangerous. True or false? _____

3. Everything you can see or touch, except _____ or _____ is a _____.

4. Vapors are formed when liquids _____ into the air.

5. The _____ the temperature, the _____ vapors will form.

6. All nail enhancement systems will form _____. Give four examples.

   a. _____

   b. _____

   c. _____

   d. _____

7. Odorless monomers do not form vapors. True or false? _____

8. Chemicals that stick two surfaces together are called _____.

9. Nail products that improve adhesion are called _____.

10. There are three types of primers used to improve adhesion of nail enhancements:

    a. _____

    b. _____

    c. _____

11. If used incorrectly, primers can eat holes in the nail plates. True or false? _____

12. Nail primers can be very corrosive to soft tissue. True or false? _____.

13. What should you wear when handling primers, adhesives, wrap resins, acrylic monomers, and UV gels?

    _____

14. The _____ tissue can be burned by corrosive, _____ primers.

15. Burning can result from _____ the natural nail, making it _____ and overly

    _____.

16. Primer should be used _____. Over-saturating the nail plate causes _____ of primer to reach the _____. This can cause _____ and _____.

17. If you are having problems with lifting, applying a _____ of primer is not the solution. Check your _____ and nail plate _____.

18. _____ or _____ primers are non-corrosive. What does this mean? _____ _____

19. Clients are not likely to become allergic to primer if _____.

20. Product vapors can cause allergic contact dermatitis. True or false? _____

21. What two factors ensure good adhesion? _____

22. You should start any nail enhancement service with a _____, _____ nail plate.

23. The risk of fingernail infections can be minimized by _____ the hands and _____ the nail plate to remove _____ and contaminants.

24. Surface _____ and _____ can _____ with product adhesion.

25. Why is it better to only dehydrate one hand at a time? _____ _____

26. Roughing up the nail improves adhesion. True or false? _____

27. Thinner _____ create a _____ for artificial nail enhancements; thicker _____ create a _____ for artificial nail enhancements.

28. Removing surface shine promotes nail adhesion. How do you remove surface shine from the nail? _____

29. Name seven things that can happen if you over-file a nail.

    a. _____

    b. _____

    c. _____

    d. _____

    e. _____

    f. _____

    g. _____

30. List five reasons for poor nail adhesion.

    a. _____

    b. _____

    c. _____

    d. _____

    e. _____

## FINGERNAIL COATINGS

31. What is a nail coating? _____

32. Name four types of nail coatings:

    a. _____

    b. _____

    c. _____

    d. _____

33. There are two main types of coatings. Name these coatings and how they work.

    a. _____

    b. _____

34. Nail polish and topcoats undergo a _____ by hardening through _____.

35. Artificial nail enhancements _____ or _____ by undergoing a _____.

36. Artificial nails or coatings are created by _____. All monomer _____ and

    _____, _____, _____, _____, and _____ work in this

    fashion.

37. What are polymers? _____. Because protein is a polymer, the _____

    that makes up the majority of the nail plate is also a _____.

38. _____ are the individual molecules that join to make the _____.

39. Define polymerization. _____

    _____.

40. Gels or no-light gels, wraps, and liquid-and-powder systems are all made from a _____, but

    _____ monomer.

41. An _____ is an ingredient that energizes molecules.

42. As rapid _____ takes place, there is _____, and the polymers become

    _____ and _____. This causes _____ of the product.

43. Chains that have had their growth halted before they were long enough to become polymers are called

    _____. They are useful in some products because they can form _____.

44. _____ create a _____ consistency in UV gels. Without _____, UV gel products

    could take up to _____, instead of _____ to harden.

45. Monomers create long chains by attaching the _____ of one monomer with the _____

    of another monomer. These are called _____.

46. Wraps and adhesive are formed by _____.

47. Simple polymer chains can be unraveled by three methods. What are they?

    a. _____

    b. _____

    c. _____

48. _____ agents strengthen simple _____ chains.

49. _____ agents are like _____ of a ladder. They make natural and artificial nails more resistant to _____ and make the nails _____, _____, and

    _____.

50. _____, _____, and _____ do not polymerize; they work strictly by

    _____.

51. The majority of ingredients in the above three products are _____ solvents. What does this

    mean? _____

52. The _____ in nail polishes, top coats, and base coats are not _____.

    This allows them to _____ quickly.

53. What is left behind after the solvents evaporate? _____

54. Because polishes do not have _____ polymers, they _____ more easily than arti-

    ficial nail enhancements.

## "BETTER FOR THE NAIL" CLAIMS

55. Certain types of artificial nail enhancement products are better for the natural nail. True or false?

    _____

56. Nurturing the nail plate and surrounding skin is the job of every _____.

57. When nail problems do arise, what are the most likely culprits?

    a. _____

    b. _____

    c. _____

58. Removing artificial nail enhancements entails soaking the fingertips in acetone. Why should you put a

    towel over your client's hands when doing this? _____

    _____.

59. All things on earth are _____ to a certain degree. Toxicity does not make a substance

    automatically unsafe, instead it means that we must learn how to use it in a _____.

# MATCHING REVIEW

*Insert the word or term that most closely fits at the left of each definition below.*

| | | |
|---|---|---|
| solvent | nonacid primers | polymerization |
| coating | corrosive | cross-linker |
| polymer | matter | evaporate |
| monomers | initiator | acid-free primer |
| primers | oligomers | simple polymer chains |
| adhesive | | |

60. _____ long chains of monomers attached from head to tail

61. _____ to change from liquid to vapor

62. _____ something that dissolves another substance

63. _____ a gigantic chain of molecules

64. _____ takes up space

65. _____ chemical that makes two surfaces stick together

66. _____ single molecules that join together to form a polymer chain

67. _____ something that energizes a molecule

68. _____ substance capable of seriously damaging skin

69. _____ substances that improve adhesion

70. _____ short chains of monomers

71. _____ does not contain acids

72. _____ does not contain methacrylic acid

73. _____ hardened film

74. _____ chemical reaction that creates polymers

75. _____ monomer that joins polymer chains together

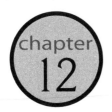
# Basics of Electricity

## INTRODUCTION

1. As a nail technician, your career heavily relies on _____.

2. Name four electrical appliances or electricity-powered products that you use as a nail technician.

   a. _____

   b. _____

   c. _____

   d. _____

3. When you see sparks fly, are you seeing electricity? _____

   _____

4. Any substance that conducts electricity is called a _____.

5. A substance that does not easily transmit electricity is called an _____ or _____.

6. List four examples of things that are poor conductors of electricity.

   a. _____

   b. _____

   c. _____

   d. _____

   e. _____

7. Name the two types of electrical current.

   a. _____ or _____

   b. _____ or _____

8. An even-flowing current that travels in only one direction is called a _____ or

   _____.

9. A rapid and interrupted current that flows in one direction and then in the opposite direction

   _____ per second is called a(n) _____ or _____.

10. Examples of devices that use direct current are _____.

11. Examples of devices that use alternating current are _____.

12. An _____ flows through a wire in much the same way as _____ flows through a hose.

13. The pressure or force that pushes the flow of electrons through a conductor is measured in _____ or _____.

14. The unit that measures the strength of an electric current is a(n) _____ or ampere.

15. What is meant by measuring the strength of an electric current? _____ _____

16. What does a higher amp rating mean? _____

17. The current in facial and scalp treatments is measured in milliamperes. What is a milliampere? _____

18. The resistance of an electric current is measured in _____.

19. The measurement of how much energy is being used in 1 second is measured in _____.

20. Unless the force or _____ is stronger than the resistance or _____, current will not flow through a _____.

21. What is a kilowatt? _____

22. The electricity in your home is measured in kilowatts per hour or _____.

23. A hair dryer can use 1000 watts of energy _____.

24. A device that is designed to blow out or melt when a wire becomes too hot from overloading the circuit with too much current is called a _____.

25. A switch that automatically interrupts or shuts off an electric circuit at the first indication of overload is called a _____. Unlike fuses, _____ do not have to be replaced, and can simply be _____.

26. What should you do when a circuit breaker shuts off? _____ _____

27. What should you do with your electrical equipment on a regular basis? _____ _____

28. What agency certifies the safety of electrical appliances? _____ or _____. What does this mean? _____

29. What are the two electrical connections of all electrical appliances? The _____ connection supplies _____ to the _____; the _____ connection completes the _____ and carries the _____ safely away to the _____.

30. Some appliances have an _____ ground for added safety. This creates a _____ path of _____, even if the first ground _____.

31. The following are rules for electrical safety. Fill in the missing words.

    a. All appliances should be _____.

    b. Read all _____ before _____.

    c. _____ appliances when not in use.

    d. Keep all _____, _____, and _____ in good repair.

    e. Never _____ a circuit by plugging in _____ appliances in one outlet.

    f. Avoid using appliances when you are in contact with _____ or _____ objects.

    g. Never clean around appliances while they are _____.

    h. Never leave a client unattended while _____ to an electrical device.

    i. Never handle electrical equipment with _____.

    j. Never touch two _____ at the same time.

    k. Keep _____ off the ground, and out of the way of client's

    _____.

    l. Electrical cords should never be allowed to become _____.

    m. Pull the _____, not the _____, when disconnecting appliances.

    n. Unless you are qualified to do so, never attempt to _____ an electrical appliance.

## Light and Heat Energy

32. What are catalysts used for? _____

33. What energy source do catalysts use? _____

34. Regardless of the source, catalysts absorb energy like a _____. They pass this energy on to an _____, and the _____ begins.

35. It is important to protect UV-curing products from all light sources because even artificial room lights can start _____ in the _____.

36. In the case of heat-curing monomers, leaving the product in a _____ car or even a sunny window can start the _____ process in the _____.

## MATCHING REVIEW

*Write in the term that most closely fits each description on the right.*

| | | |
|---|---|---|
| electric current | amp or ampere | volt |
| insulator | direct current | ohm |
| electricity | alternating current | circuit breaker |
| milliampere | conductor | kilowatt |

37. _____ 1/1000 of an amp

38. _____ rapid and interrupted current

39. _____ switch that automatically shuts off an electric circuit

40. _____ form of energy

41. _____ current that travels in one direction

42. _____ poor conductor of electricity

43. _____ measures the resistance of an electric current

44. _____ measures the flow of electrons forward through a conductor

45. _____ 1000 watts

46. _____ measures the strength of an electric current

47. _____ any substance that readily conducts electricity

48. _____ flow of electricity along a conductor

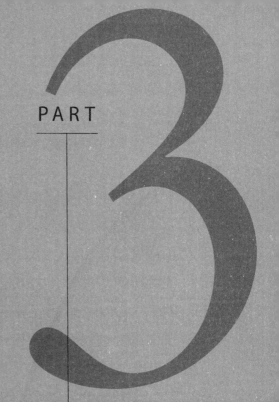

# NAIL CARE

Date _____

Rating _____

Text Pages 196–235

# Manicuring

## INTRODUCTION

1. What type of bulb should you have for your manicuring lamp? _____
   _____

2. The trash receptacle next to your workstation should ideally be made of _____ and have a
   _____ lid.

3. How do you hold a wooden pusher? _____

4. How do you hold a metal pusher? _____

5. What is the spoon end of a metal pusher used for? _____

6. Why should you dull any rough edges on your metal pusher? _____
   _____

7. List the grit range for fine, medium, and coarse nail abrasives.

   a. Coarse _____

   b. Medium _____

   c. Fine _____

8. Coarse nail files are more _____ and should never be used on _____.

9. Medium-grit abrasives are used to _____ and _____ surfaces.

10. Fine-grit abrasives are used for _____, _____, and _____ very fine scratches on
    the nail plate.

11. How do you bevel a nail? _____
    _____

12. Many abrasive boards and buffers can be sanitized and disinfected. True or false? _____

13. Never store your abrasives or other implements in a plastic bag or other sealed container. Why?
    _____

14. Nippers should never be used to remove _____.

15. How should you hold a nipper? Place your _____ on _____ and _____
    on the _____, with your _____ on the _____ to help
    _____ the blade.

16. What causes hardened tissue around the proximal nail fold? _____

17. How do you treat this hardened tissue? _____
_____

18. **Matching.** *Match the names of the tools and equipment with the correct descriptions on the right.*

_____ 1. fingerbowl

_____ 2. disinfection container

_____ 3. client's arm cushion

_____ 4. wipe container

_____ 5. supply tray

_____ 6. UV/electric nail polish dryer

_____ 7. wooden pusher

_____ 8. metal pusher

_____ 9. medium grit

_____ 10. coarse grit

_____ 11. fine grit

_____ 12. tweezer

_____ 13. nipper

_____ 14. nail brush

_____ 15. applicator brush

_____ 16. three-way buffer

_____ 17. nail clippers

_____ 18. chamois

A. used to scrub the nails

B. used to smooth and refine surfaces

C. multi-purpose tool

D. used to trim away tags of dead skin

E. 240 or higher grit

F. can be reused if properly sanitized and disinfected

G. closed container for cotton balls

H. replaces the chamois

I. used to shorten the nail plate

J. disposable instrument to push back cuticles

K. 8" x 12" cushion

L. speeds up the nail-polish drying process

M. not to be used on natural nails

N. bowl for soaking client's fingers

O. soft leather used to shine the natural nail

P. durable, easy to clean tray for cosmetics

Q. container with a lid that is big enough to fully immerse implements in disinfectant solution

R. used to push back the eponychium

19. A brush or applicator must be _____ of after a _____ use, except when it is used in a _____ solution. Examples of _____ solutions follow:

a. _____

b. _____

c. _____

d. _____

e. _____

f. _____

g. _____

20. _____ and _____ are solvents commonly used in polish removers.

21. Non-acetone polish removers generally contain _____ or _____.

22. _____ removers are used to remove _____ from _____ enhancements because they do not _____ the _____ as quickly as _____ removers.

23. Name three important benefits of nail creams or penetrating nail oils.

    a. _____

    b. _____

    c. _____

24. Products that are designed to _____ and _____ dead tissue from the nail plate are called

    _____.

25. Cuticle removers can be very _____ and _____ to living tissue because they contain

    _____ amounts of _____ ingredients.

26. _____ percent _____ and _____ hydroxide are key active ingredients in

    many _____.

27. Three symptoms of over-exposure of cuticle removers include:

    a. _____

    b. _____

    c. _____

28. Lightening agents in nail bleach are generally _____, or some other _____ agent.

29. Nail bleaches are considered _____ and should have _____ skin contact.

30. A generic term for any solvent-based colored film applied to the nail plate for cosmetic purposes is

    _____.

31. Other terms for the above product include _____, _____, and _____. These are

    _____ and _____ indicate a _____ kind of formulation.

32. Nitrocellulose is a _____ material.

33. When the solvents _____ in nail polish, a _____ is left on the _____.

34. What determines the drying time of polish?

    a. _____

    b. _____

    c. _____

35. Nail polish, base coat, and top coat are highly flammable. True or false? _____

36. The base coat has two purposes. What are they?

    a. _____.

    b. _____.

# MATCHING REVIEW

*Insert the correct product name for each definition. Note: a product may be appropriate for more than one description.*

base coat
soap
nail bleach
non–acetone
formaldehyde
ethyl acetate
paraffin treatment

nail polish
pumice powder
nail oil/cream
hardener
protein hardener
top coat

nitrocellulose
cuticle remover
acetone
solvent
nylon
dimethyl urea

37. _____ clear polish and collagen formula used to harden the nail plate

38. _____ solvent used in nail polish

39. _____ used to clean hands before the service begins

40. _____ containing ethyl acetate or methyl ethyl ketone

41. _____ hardens by cross-linking the keratin strands of the nail plate

42. _____ removes yellow surface discolorations or stains

43. _____ softens hands, speeds up penetration of cream or lotion

44. _____ hardens nails, but can have adverse skin reactions

45. _____ relies on resins to anchor polish

46. _____ nail hardener that adds cross-links without adverse skin reactions

47. _____ seals in moisture and softens cuticles

48. _____ typically contains acrylic and film formers

49. _____ loosens dead tissue from the nail plate

50. _____ solvent used to remove nail polish

51. _____ prevents staining caused by colored nail polish

52. _____ reinforcing fiber that strengthens and coats the nail plate

53. _____ usually has 2% to 5% sodium or potassium hydroxide and moisturizers

54. _____ enhances flexibility of the nail plate

55. _____ mild abrasive used to smooth and polish the nail plate

56. _____ sticky product that enhances adhesion of nail polish

57. _____ improves the durability of weak or thin nails

58. _____ film-forming substance

59. _____ lacquer, varnish, or enamel

# BASIC TABLE SETUP

60. List the steps of a basic table setup.

a. _____.

b. _____.

c.  Fill disinfectant container.

d.  _____.

e.  Arrange abrasives.

f.  _____.

g.  _____.

h.  Place polishes.

i.  _____.

61.  If you are right-handed, your polishes should be placed on the _____ side of your table.

62.  When choosing the length and shape of the nail, you should take the following into consideration:

a.  _____

b.  _____

c.  _____

d.  _____

e.  _____

63.  Identify the five basic nail shapes below.

a.  _____

b.  _____

c.  _____

d.  _____

e.  _____

64.  Male clients generally prefer round–shaped nails because they _____ the natural _____ of the nail tip.

65.  An _____ shape is the most _____ nail shape.

66.  Thin hands and nail beds look best with _____ nails.

67.  The weakest nail shape is a _____ nail; the _____ nail shape is sturdy because the width of the nail is not altered.

68.  List the procedure that you should follow when blood is drawn during a manicure.

a.  Put on _____.

b.  Apply _____.

c.  _____ bleeding.

d.  _____.

e.  Discard used materials.

f.  Clean _____ and disinfect _____.

g.  _____.

69. List the procedures that you should follow for pre-service sanitation.

    a. _____ implements.

    b. Rinse _____ in water.

    c. Immerse _____.

    d. Wash hands with _____.

    e. _____.

    f. Follow approved _____ procedure.

    g. _____.

    h. _____.

    i. Prepare client's _____.

    j. Refill _____.

    k. Use hand _____.

70. What should you always do in front of clients prior to their services? _____

_____

71. List the proper post-service steps.

    a. _____.

    b. _____.

    c. Promote _____.

    d. Clean _____.

    e. Disinfect _____.

    f. Record _____.

## BASIC MANICURE

72. By breaking your procedures down into _____, it is easy to keep track of what you are doing.

They are _____, _____, and _____.

73. Once your client is physically at your workstation, list the steps that you should do before beginning the

nail service.

    a. Greet client.

    b. Have client remove _____ and place in a _____ place.

    c. Ask client to _____.

    d. Perform _____ and fill out _____.

74. When beginning a manicure, always start with the hand that is not the client's _____ hand. If the

client is _____-handed, you should begin with the _____ hand.

75. Where should you begin working on the hand? _____

76. Why should you always file the nails before soaking them? _____

_____

77. When polish residue is in the nail fold or cuticle area, what should you do? _____

_____

_____

78. When removing cuticle that is tightly adhered to the nail plate with a pusher, use _____

motions.

79. Why should you gently clean under the free edge? _____

_____

80. Applying too much force or pressure to the eponychium can damage what? _____

81. Never shake your _____. Shaking causes _____ to form and makes your applica-

tion _____ and _____.

82. Nail strengthener/hardener should be applied before the _____.

83. Nail bleaches and cuticle removers can cause what? _____

84. List the four coats of polish that are applied to a client's nails during a manicure service.

    a. _____

    b. _____

    c. _____

    d. _____

85. When shaping the nail, you should always file from the _____ of the nail.

## Manicure Service

86. List and explain the steps of a basic manicure service.

    a. Remove polish.

    b. _____.

    c. _____.

    d. Clean nails.

    e. _____.

    f. _____.

    g. _____.

    h. Clip away _____ of skin.

    i. _____.

    j. _____.

    k. _____.

    l. _____.

m. _____ .

n. Bevel nails.

o. _____ .

p. _____ .

q. Choose a color.

r. _____ .

87. Name and describe the five types of polish application.

   a. _____ .

   b. _____ .

   c. _____ .

   d. _____ .

   e. _____ .

88. What does a slim-line or _____ nail polish application accomplish? _____

   _____

89. What is the advantage of a free edge or hairline tip application? _____

90. How can you disguise pitting or striations in the nail? _____

91. What is the difference between a French manicure and American manicure? _____

   _____

92. What are the four steps of a French or American manicure?

   a. _____

   b. _____

   c. _____

   d. _____

## CONDITIONING OIL MANICURE

93. When should you recommend a conditioning oil manicure? _____

   _____

94. List the steps that you should do when performing a conditioning oil manicure.

   a. Perform pre-service sanitation and table set up.

   b. Begin manicure.

   c. _____ .

   d. _____ .

   e. _____ .

   f. Apply lotion

   g. _____ .

h. _____.

i. Remove tags of dead skin.

j. Repeat on other hand.

k. _____.

l. _____.

m. _____.

n. Complete manicure post-service.

95. When performing a man's manicure, follow the steps outlined for a _____ or _____, but replace the colored polish step with either _____ or with _____.

96. What is paraffin? _____

97. Why is a paraffin treatment beneficial to the skin? _____

98. What are the contraindications for a paraffin wax treatment? _____

_____

99. List the steps for a paraffin wax treatment before the manicure.

a. _____.

b. Check client's hands to ensure that they have no open wounds.

c. _____.

d. Test the temperature of the wax.

e. _____.

f. _____

_____.

g. _____.

h. _____.

i. Repeat this procedure on the other hand.

j. _____.

k. _____.

l. _____.

m. _____.

100. When should you do a paraffin wax treatment during a manicure? _____

_____

## HAND AND ARM MASSAGE

101. Hand-and-arm massage can be done with any _____, but it is always done in a _____.

102. A massage done during a manicure should have _____ and _____ movements.

103. A massage should be done after the _____ is complete, and before the
     _____ application.

104. List and describe three basic movements used during a massage.

     a. _____

     b. _____

     c. _____

105. List two things that massage does for clients: _____.

106. While giving a hand-and-arm massage, practice sound ergonomics by never _____ toward your
     client.

107. What medical conditions are contraindicative of massage?

     a. _____

     b. _____

     c. _____

## SPA MANICURE

108. A spa manicure requires a basic knowledge of _____.

109. List three characteristics of a spa manicure.

     a. _____

     b. _____

     c. _____

110. All spa manicures include an _____ step to smooth the skin and enhance
     _____ of products.

111. Additional techniques and steps that can be included in a spa manicure follow:

     a. Aromatic paraffin treatments

     b. _____

     c. _____

     d. _____

     e. _____

112. What is aromatherapy? _____

# Pedicuring

## INTRODUCTION

1. List the five basic steps of a pedicure procedure.

   a. _____

   b. _____

   c. _____

   d. _____

   e. _____

2. Because clients will have different needs, you should tailor your pedicure service to meet the needs of your entire clientele. True or False _____

3. What type of shoes should clients wear to a pedicure appointment? _____.

   Why? _____

4. Why should clients not shave their legs 24 hours before a pedicure service? _____

   _____

5. Toenail clippers can have either _____ or _____ jaws.

6. A nail rasp smoothes the _____; it is designed to only file _____.

7. Foot files and paddles are _____ than those designed for the hands.

8. A major advantage of the diamond-cut file is it _____.

9. The curette is used to remove debris from the _____ and _____.

## PEDICURE EQUIPMENT AND MATERIALS

10. **Matching.** *Match the terms on the left with correct descriptions on the right. Note: Some terms will have more than one appropriate description.*

   _____ 1. foot bath          A. keeps toes apart

   _____ 2. toenail clipper    B. designed to file in one direction

   _____ 3. pedicuring stool   C. should have an armrest and be comfortable

   _____ 4. foot file          D. loosens the nail's cuticle

   _____ 5. foot powder        E. shortens the length of the toenails

   _____ 6. toe separators     F. disposable paper foot slippers

_____ 7. pedicuring station    G. keeps feet dry after a pedicure

_____ 8. foot lotion    H. filled with warm soapy water

_____ 9. client's chair    I. includes two chairs and a footrest

_____ 10. pedicure slippers    J. used during a foot massage

_____ 11. nail rasp    K. nail technician's low stool

                           L. removes ingrown toenails

                           M. smoothes calluses

11. Besides standard manicuring implements, list the equipment, implements, and supplies needed to do a basic pedicure service.

     a. _____

     b. _____

     c. _____

     d. _____

     e. _____

     f. _____

     g. _____

     h. _____

     i. _____

     j. _____

12. Like a manicure, a pedicure involves a _____ service: _____
_____.

13. What do you do if you notice an infection or inflammation on your client's feet? _____
_____.

14. Why is it important to have your client fill out a consultation form prior to a pedicure? _____
_____
_____

15. List the steps for a standard pedicure procedure.

     a. Remove shoes and socks.

     b. _____.

     c. _____.

     d. _____.

     e. Clip nails.

     f. _____.

     g. _____.

     h. Rinse foot.

i. _____.

j. _____.

k. _____.

l. _____.

m. _____.

n. _____.

o. Massage foot.

p. Repeat steps a through j on other foot.

q. _____.

r. _____.

16. List the six steps of a pedicure post-service procedure.

a. _____.

b. Advise client.

c. _____.

d. _____.

e. _____.

f. If used as part of this service, _____ manicure table.

## FOOT MASSAGE

17. Define massage. _____
_____

18. What are the names of the three basic hand movements used in a pedicure massage? Describe them.

a. _____ Compression movements such as _____, _____, and _____ that _____ muscles and tendons

b. _____ A rapid succession of _____ movements using the _____ of the hands

c. Effleurage. _____ or _____ strokes used to _____ muscles and improve _____ to the small, surface capillaries

19. When giving a leg-and-foot massage, practice good ergonomics by:

a. Keeping your _____ straight.

b. Not _____ or leaning _____ to reach your client's feet.

c. Sit in a _____ and _____ position.

20. What three medical conditions would preclude receiving a foot massage?

a. _____

b. _____

c. _____

21. Basic pedicure products are available in four general categories:

    a. _____

    b. _____

    c. _____

    d. _____

22. In terms of cleaning and deodorizing the feet, _____ soaps _____more effective than soaps that do not make this claim.

23. _____ set the stage for a pedicure service.

24. _____ salts are one of the ingredients often found in foot soaks. This product has _____ that are believed to be _____ to the skin.

25. When soaking the feet during a pedicure, the water temperature must not exceed _____.

26. Leaving hooks or sharp points on the sides of the big toenails can cause _____.

27. When should you use an abrasive foot scrub? _____

28. Name five products commonly used as exfoliating agents in pedicure scrubs.

    a. _____

    b. _____

    c. _____

    d. _____

    e. _____

29. What is a massage preparation? _____

30. Add _____ to a massage preparation for its _____ and _____ effects.

31. _____ are used to _____ hardened tissue.

32. _____, _____, _____, _____, and beneficial extracts are typically found in foot masques.

33. Name at least four add-on products that are used to enhance and expedite the pedicure experience.

    a. _____

    b. _____

    c. _____

    d. _____

## MATCHING REVIEW

*Insert the word or term that most closely fits each definition below.*

| | | |
|---|---|---|
| closed toe | friction | straight across |
| curved nail rasp | tapotement | effleurage |
| open-toed | toenail clippers | foot bath |
| pedicure | toe separators | foot file |
| pedicuring stool | foot powder | petrissage |
| Dead Sea salts | callus softener | aromatherapy |
| pedicure cart | pedicure throne | |

34. _____ shortens the length of the nail

35. _____ relaxing massage movement

36. _____ includes trimming, shaping, massage, and polishing the toenails

37. _____ removes dry skin or callus growth

38. _____ helps to soften and smooth hardened skin

39. _____ kneading massage movement

40. _____ shape or direction into which toenails should be filed

41. _____ type of shoes client should wear for a pedicure appointment

42. _____ keep toes apart during a pedicure

43. _____ a light tapping massage movement

44. _____ filled with soapy water.

45. _____ deep rubbing massage movements such as thumb and fist twist compression

46. _____ the ultimate pedicure station

47. _____ keeps feet dry after a pedicure

48. _____ files in one direction

49. _____ a cart on wheels with drawers to hold pedicure supplies

50. _____ essential oils with beneficial properties

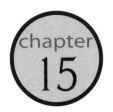

# Electric Filing

## INTRODUCTION

1. What do the letters AEFM stand for? _____
   _____

2. List the different types of electric files and rate their power and suitability for nail services.

   a. _____

   b. _____

   c. _____

3. Because the motor is in the hand piece, all professional electric files are called _____.

4. What does the _____ of a hobby tool do to the nails?

   a. _____.

   b. _____.

   c. _____.

5. What features should you look for in an electric nail file?

   a. _____

   b. _____

   c. _____

   d. _____

   e. _____

   f. _____

   g. _____

   h. _____

6. Revolutions per minute or (RPMs) indicates the _____
   _____.

7. RPM capacity of nail files can vary from _____ to _____.

8. Torque is _____. The more powerful the machine, the _____.

9. Lighter machines have _____. They can do the same thing as _____,
   but _____.

10. You should never use an electric file until you have received _____ and had plenty of _____.

11. Your electric file will be in good working order for many years if _____

_____ .

## CHOOSING BITS

12. Bits that are balanced while spinning are called _____ .

13. A bit that is not concentric is _____ .

14. If the edges of a bit are sharp, what should you do? _____

_____

15. How do you measure grit? _____

16. How are carbide bits measured? _____

17. What are diamond bits? _____

_____ .

18. Higher quality diamond bits have more _____ in construction because each particle on every bit

is cut the _____ and then adhered to medical stainless steel.

19. Carbide bits come in a variety of shapes, sizes, grits, and metals. Carbide bits have _____ that are

cut at an angle. Instead of chipping like _____ , carbide bits _____ as

they file.

20. Name and explain two basic kinds of carbide bits.

a. _____ .

b. _____

_____ .

21. What do Swiss carbides do? _____

22. What are buffing bits? They are made out of _____ , _____ materials such as

_____ , _____ _____ , or _____ .

23. Foot calluses are smoothed with _____ , _____ , and _____ particles.

24. To attach nail jewelry, a _____ .

25. How do you disinfect bits?

a. Clean the bit.

b. _____ .

c. _____ .

d. Store in a _____ .

26. List the three ways to clean or sanitize a bit before disinfecting.

a. _____ .

b. _____ .

c. _____ .

27. For better control, use a _____ during filing.

28. Balance your arm by _____. This keeps the _____ secure and _____ movement during filing.

29. How do you hold the handpiece? _____

30. The bit should be _____ and _____ with the table.

31. You know your drill speed is too slow when it _____.

32. When rebalancing nails, smooth the old product in the growth area with a _____ bit.

33. To repair cracks, slowly bevel a trench with the body of the bit by _____ _____.

34. The key to finishing the nails without leaving scratches is to _____.

35. Unlike hand-held abrasives, _____ is the coarsest grit for an electric file.

36. The use of _____ can reduce heat and hold dust to the surface of the bit.

37. Lift the buffing bit _____ and _____ to avoid overheating the nail and possibly burning your client.

38. _____ can dramatically enhance the shine of nails when used in conjunction with a(n) _____.

39. _____ have the smallest particles of dust. When using _____, an appropriate dust mask should always be worn.

40. Diamond bits create heavier particles that _____ fly high into the air.

41. _____ and _____ bits shave the surface of the product, creating heavier particles that are _____ at the table.

42. What causes heat to build up on the nail?

    a. _____

    b. _____

    c. _____

    d. _____

43. To dramatically reduce heat on the nail:

    a. _____.

    b. _____.

    c. _____.

    d. _____.

44. What is grabbing? _____

45. What causes grabbing?

    a. _____.

    b. _____.

46. How can grabbing be avoided?

    a. _____ .

    b. _____ .

    c. _____ .

47. What causes rings of fire?

    a. _____

    b. _____

48. How can you avoid causing rings of fire?

    a. _____ .

    b. _____ .

    c. _____ .

## PRODUCT BREAKDOWN

49. After several weeks products can become brittle. When this happens, _____ can occur.

List some potential causes of microshattering.

    a. _____

    b. _____

    c. _____

    d. _____

    e. _____

    f. _____

    g. _____

50. List possible solutions to microshattering.

    a. _____

    b. _____

    c. _____

    d. _____

    e. _____

    f. _____

    g. _____

    h. _____

## MATCHING REVIEW

*Match the words or terms with the correct explanations, descriptions, or definitions.*

bit
torque
non-concentric bit
sanders or sleeves
diamond bits
variable-speed foot pedal

crosscut carbides
flutes
rings of fire
closed casings
hobby and craft
carbide bits

Swiss carbide bits
RPMs
pedicure bits
grit
forward and reverse

51. _____ attachment that actually does the filing

52. _____ imbalanced bit that wobbles or vibrates

53. _____ long, slender cuts or grooves found on carbide and Swiss carbide bits

54. _____ can be used to file both directions

55. _____ number of abrasive particles per square inch

56. _____ slot-free design to prevent dust from contaminating the motor

57. _____ varying types of metals, shapes, sizes, and grits

58. _____ made of paper, non-cutting bit called a mandrel

59. _____ speed of the machine

60. _____ works like the accelerator on a car

61. _____ grooves carved into the nail

62. _____ made of diamond, sapphire, and ruby particles

63. _____ shave the surface as they file

64. _____ power of the machine

65. _____ designed for use on glass, wood, and ceramics

66. _____ necessary for left-handed technicians

67. _____ chip the surface of the product

Date _____

Rating _____

Text Pages 274–293

# Nail Tips, Wraps, and No-Light Gels

## INTRODUCTION

1. What is a nail tip? _____

2. What are nail tips used for?

    a. _____

    b. _____

3. Without an overlay, a nail tip will _____.

4. What are overlays? _____

    _____

5. Nail tips require special products and implements. What are they? What are they used for?

    a. _____

    b. _____

    c. _____

    d. _____

6. The _____ is a depression that serves as the point of contact with the nail plate. Nail tips come

    with three different variations of this design feature. What are they?

    a. _____

    b. _____

    c. _____

7. Label the half well, full well, and the position stop on the

    nail tip illustration.

    1. _____

    2. _____

    3. _____

8. The nail tip covers _____ or less of the natural nail plate.

9. To ensure a perfect fit and shape for every client, nail tips are available in many _____.

10. Describe a prefect nail tip fit. _____

11. Besides not being aesthetically pleasing, what two things can happen when a nail tip is narrower than the nail plate? _____

12. If you do not have a tip that provides a perfect fit, what should you do? _____

_____

13. To save time blending the tip after it is applied, what should you do? _____

_____

14. When applying tips, you should use the _____, _____, and _____ procedure. Explain these three steps.

    a. _____

    _____

    b. _____

    c. _____

15. What tools are used to trim nail tips to the desired length? _____

## NAIL TIP APPLICATION

16. List the nail tip application procedure.

    a. Complete pre-service _____ and _____ procedure.

    b. Add these items to your standard manicuring table setup: _____,

    _____, _____, _____, and

    _____.

    c. Greet client and ask her to _____.

    d. Check for nail disorders.

    e. Remove _____.

    f. _____.

    g. Remove _____.

    h. _____.

    i. _____.

    j. _____.

    k. _____.

    l. _____.

    m. _____.

    n. _____.

    o. _____.

    p. Proceed with desired nail enhancement service.

17. List the three most important steps of the post-service procedure, when the client has received a nail tip, nail wrap, or no-light gel service.

    a. _____.

    b. _____.

    c. _____.

18. List and describe how to safely remove a nail tip or fabric nail wrap.

    a. _____.

    b. _____.

    c. _____.

19. When a client has nail tips and/or nail wraps, what type of polish remover should you use?

    _____

20. Use a _____ abrasive to lightly buff the nail plates and remove shine.

## NAIL WRAPS

21. What is a nail wrap? _____

    _____

22. What are pre-cut nail wraps? _____

    _____

23. What is a nail wrap used for?

    a. _____

    b. _____

24. Fabric wraps are made from three different fabrics. What are they? Describe their unique characteristics.

    a. _____.

    b. _____.

    c. _____.

    _____.

25. What are the three biggest challenges associated with linen wraps?

    a. _____.

    b. _____.

    c. _____.

26. Where do you apply nail adhesive when affixing fabric to the nail? _____

27. You should always leave a _____ margin between the fabric and the _____ and

    _____.

28. What two things can occur when you do not keep adhesive off the skin?

    a. _____

    b. _____

29. How should you apply wrap resin? _____

30. Why should you use a plastic sheet as part of a fabric wrap service?

    a. _____.

    b. _____.

    _____.

31. How do you remove traces of oil prior to polishing the nails? _____

    _____.

32. In addition to the materials used for a basic manicure set-up, what additional items do you need to per-

    form a fabric wrap service?

    a. _____

    b. _____

    c. _____

    d. _____

    e. _____

    f. _____

    g. _____

    h. _____

    i. _____

33. List the steps in a nail wrap application.

    a. Perform a complete pre-service _____ and _____ procedure.

    b. Do a standard table set-up plus all implements and supplies needed to perform a fabric wrap service.

    c. Greet client and ask her to _____.

    d. Check for nail disorders.

    e. Remove _____.

    f. _____.

    g. _____.

    h. Remove _____.

    i. _____.

    j. Apply nail tips, if desired.

    k. Cut fabric.

    l. _____.

    m. _____.

    n. _____.

    o. _____.

    p. _____.

q. Apply second coat of wrap resin.

r. _____.

s. _____.

t. _____.

u. Remove traces of oil.

v. _____.

34. You should maintain fabric wraps _____.

35. How is the protocol for a 2-week maintenance visit different than the initial fabric wrap application?

a. Instead of applying the fabric to the entire nail, you _____,

followed by _____ on the freshly applied product.

b. _____ is then applied to the entire nail, followed by an _____.

36. What should be done at the 4-week service? How is it different from the initial fabric wrap application?

a. Instead of applying fabric to the entire nail, you _____,

allowing it to slightly _____.

b. You apply wrap resin to the _____, followed by an application of

_____ on the freshly applied product.

c. _____ is then applied to _____, followed by _____.

## REPAIRS WITH FABRIC WRAPS

37. You can use fabric to create a _____ to strengthen a weak point, or a _____

to repair a break.

38. Describe how the fabric is applied to reinforce a weak point. _____

_____

39. Describe how fabric is used to repair a break or crack. _____

_____

## NO-LIGHT GELS

40. What is a no-light gel? _____

41. Why is it called "no-light" gel? _____

42. What cures the gel? _____

43. No-light gels can be used alone or with _____ or _____ fabrics. Layering no-light

gel with these fabrics creates a _____ nail.

44. Besides your basic manicuring set-up, you will need the following products and implements:

   a. _____

   b. _____

   c. _____

   d. _____

   e. _____

45. List the standard procedures for applying no-light gel products. Remember to always read the manufacturer's directions for specific application steps with a particular product or system.

   a. Complete the no-light gel application pre-service.

   b. Remove existing polish.

   c. _____.

   d. _____.

   e. _____.

   f. Apply nail tips, if desired.

   g. _____.

   h. Apply no-light gel.

   i. _____.

   j. Repeat steps g, h, and i on the right hand.

   k. Apply second coat of no-light gel, if required.

   l. Shape and refine nails.

   m. _____.

   n. _____.

   o. _____.

   p. _____.

   q. Apply nail polish.

   r. Complete no-light gel application post-service.

## NO-LIGHT GEL AND FIBERGLASS/SILK FABRIC

46. No-light gels and fiberglass/silk fabric applications create a _____ nail enhancement.

47. With this type of enhancement, fabric is used between the _____.

48. List the steps for a no-light gel and fiberglass/silk fabric application.

   a. Prepare fabric strips that are no greater than _____.

   b. Using a new wooden pusher, place two sections of material _____ to form an _____.

   c. _____.

# MATCHING REVIEW

*Match the following words or terms with the description or definition that most closely fits.*

| | | |
|---|---|---|
| no–light gel | repair patch | fabric wraps |
| buffer block | nail tip | silk |
| nail wraps | tip cutter | stress strip |
| fiberglass | linen | activator |
| accelerator | | |

49. _____ a piece of fabric cut to cover a crack or break

50. _____ does not require UV light to cure

51. _____ nail-size pieces of cloth that are bonded to the top of the nail plate

52. _____ a strip of fabric used to strengthen a weak point in the nail

53. _____ thick, strong fabric

54. _____ cures no–light gels

55. _____ light-weight, rectangular abrasives

56. _____ very thin synthetic mesh with a loose weave

57. _____ hardens fiberglass wraps

58. _____ used to shorten nail tips

59. _____ made with ABS or tenite acetate polymer

60. _____ becomes transparent when adhesive is applied

61. _____ silk, linen, and fiberglass

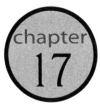

chapter

17

# Acrylic (Methacrylate) Nail Enhancements

## INTRODUCTION

1. Define acrylic (methacrylate) nails. _____

2. Nearly all ingredients used for artificial nail enhancements come from the _____ family.

3. _____, a branch of the _____, are used in _____

   enhancement systems.

4. Liquid and powder enhancements are created by combining _____ and

   _____ .

5. "Mono" means _____ and "poly" means _____ .

6. What makes up the majority of the liquid portion of acrylic nail enhancements? _____

   _____

7. What makes up the majority of the powder portion of acrylic nail enhancements? _____

   _____

8. Why are catalysts and initiators included in liquid monomer?

   a. Catalysts _____ .

   b. Initiators _____ .

9. What is the initiator in acrylic powder? _____

10. Different amounts of BPO are used in different products. True or false? _____ .

11. Combining different brands of products to form a nail enhancement can lead to _____

    and possible _____ due to _____ .

12. Besides ensuring a good cure, what do different additives provide for different acrylic nail products?

    a. _____

    b. _____

    c. _____

    d. _____

13. What is a mix ratio? _____

14. A _____ is created from equal amounts of liquid and powder.

15. A medium bead is generally the _____ when working with monomer liquids and polymer powders. It consists of _____.

16. The _____ and _____ of the nail enhancement are dependent on having the appropriate mix ratio.

17. Brittleness and/or discoloration are caused by what? _____

18. Weakened acrylic (methacrylate) nail enhancements can be caused by _____.

19. Hand sanitizers cannot remove _____. They only _____.

20. What product removes surface moisture and tiny amounts of oil left on the natural nail plate?

    _____

21. How should you apply acid nail primer? _____

    _____

22. Using too much product may cause the acid primer to _____.

23. How many nails should you be able to treat before re-dipping the brush in the primer? _____

24. Nail forms are available in the following materials:

    a. _____

    b. _____

    c. _____

25. All forms are disposable except those made from _____.

26. What nail enhancement product can cause serious, and sometimes irreversible damage to the skin and eyes? _____

27. To obtain maximum shelf life, how should your nail adhesives be handled?

    a. _____

    b. _____

    c. _____

    d. _____ between _____.

28. _____ are used to hold monomer liquid and polymer powder during the application process.

29. To minimize evaporation of the monomer into the air, these dishes _____.

30. Why should you never pour any unused monomer liquid back into the original product container?

    _____

    _____

31. On a daily basis, check your nail primer to ensure that it is _____, and has no _____. Contaminants can _____.

32. Sable hair makes _____.

33. _____ and _____ brushes do not pick up enough monomer liquid or

_____ .

34. Safely _____ and _____ liquid and powder nail enhancements requires that you wear

three protective devices. What are they? Why should you wear them?

a. _____

b. _____

c. _____

_____

35. What grit nail abrasives should you use to remove shine from the nail plate? _____

36. Select a medium grit _____ for _____ and _____ .

37. A fine buffer _____ should be used for final buffing. A three-way buffer is used to

_____ when _____ .

38. A 180 grit is usually coarse enough to _____ .

39. You should never use a coarser _____ abrasive on a freshly applied enhancement product.

40. It takes _____ for an acrylic (methacrylate) nail enhancement to reach ultimate strength.

41. How do you apply a disposable nail form? List the steps:

a. _____

b. _____

c. _____

d. _____

e. _____

42. How many dappen dishes do you need if you are using two colors of polymer powder? _____

_____

43. Describe the best way to dip your brush into the monomer liquid and pick up a bead of product from

the polymer powder.

a. Dip the brush in the _____ and wipe _____ to

remove the excess.

b. Dip the tip of the same brush into the _____ and _____ .

44. Never allow your brush to touch the _____ area of the nail until you apply the

_____ on the area. Why? _____

45. List the order and where these acrylic (methacrylate) beads should be placed.

a. Place the first bead of product _____ .

b. Place the second bead of product _____ .

c. Place a third smaller bead _____ .

46. When doing a pink-and-white enhancement service:

    a. The first bead is _____.

    b. The second bead is _____.

    c. The third bead is _____

47. _____ and _____ the product to spread it evenly over the nail plate.

48. Glide the brush over the nail to _____.

49. For a more natural looking nail, the product near the _____, _____, and _____ must be thin.

50. How should you discard used monomer liquid? _____

    _____

51. List the steps involved in an acrylic (methacrylate) nail enhancement pre-service.

    a. Set up your standard manicuring table. _____

    b. Greet client and ask her to _____

    _____.

    c. Perform a client consultation and note _____ and _____ on a client consultation form.

52. List the steps involved in an acrylic (methacrylate) nail enhancement service.

    a. _____.

    b. _____.

    c. Remove oily shine from natural nail.

    d. _____.

    e. Position nail form.

    f. Apply nail primer.

    g. _____.

    h. Dip brush in monomer liquid.

    i. _____.

    j. _____.

    k. Shape free edge.

    l. Place second bead of product.

    m. _____.

    n. _____.

    o. Apply product to remaining nails.

    p. _____.

    q. _____.

    r. Buff nail enhancements.

s. _____.

t. Apply hand cream and massage hand and arm.

u. _____.

v. _____.

53. List the steps that you should follow as part of the acrylic _____ nail post-service.

a. _____.

b. _____.

c. _____.

d. _____.

e. _____.

f. _____.

g. _____.

54. Describe the procedure for acrylic (methacrylate) nail enhancements over tips or natural nails. How does it differ from an acrylic (methacrylate) nail enhancement service? _____

_____

55. What is a nail rebalance? A method for maintaining the _____, _____, and _____ of the _____.

56. How often should clients wearing acrylic nail enhancements have a rebalance service? _____ What does this depend on? _____.

57. Explain why nippers should not be used to loosen nail enhancement product.

_____

58. How is a rebalance service performed?

a. Complete acrylic (methacrylate) nail enhancement application pre-service).

b. _____.

c. _____.

d. _____.

e. _____.

f. _____.

g. _____.

h. _____.

i. _____.

j. _____.

k. _____.

l. _____.

m. _____.

n. _____.

o. _____.

p. _____.

q. _____.

r. _____.

s. _____.

t. _____.

u. _____.

v. _____.

59. When shaping nail enhancements during a rebalance service, make sure to taper the nail shape toward

the _____, _____, and _____, thinning all edges.

60. If you are using a pink-and-white product application, apply the _____ acrylic (methacrylate)

first, to re-establish the _____.

61. When lightly tapped with a nailbrush handle, nails make a _____ sound when they are com-

pletely cured.

62. Describe and explain how to repair a nail crack for acrylic nail enhancements.

a. _____.

b. _____.

c. _____.

d. _____.

e. _____.

f. _____.

g. _____.

h. _____.

i. _____.

j. _____.

k. _____.

l. _____.

m. _____.

n. _____.

o. _____.

p. _____.

q. _____.

r. _____.

s. _____.

63. To remove a crack, file a _____ into the crack, or smooth it until it is _____ with the nail enhancement.

64. If a crack is big, use a _____ for _____.

65. _____ and _____ acrylic into the crack.

66. Detail how to safely remove acrylic nail enhancements.

   a. _____

   _____.

   b. _____.

   c. _____.

   d. _____.

   e. _____.

67. Gently _____ softened acrylic material with a _____.

68. Never use _____ to pry off acrylic material because it will _____.

69. After nail enhancements have been removed, why do the nail plates appear to be thinner? *Circle the right answer.*

   a. The natural nails are damaged and must completely grow out.

   b. They have been deprived of oxygen and will take time to regenerate.

   c. They contain excess water that will evaporate within 24 hours.

70. Buff the natural nail after removing the artificial enhancements to _____ _____. Use a fine _____ or higher buffer.

71. Odorless acrylics rely on _____ that have a _____.

72. In general, a _____ ratio should be used for odorless acrylic products.

73. A dry mix looks like a _____ bead on your brush.

74. The tacky layer of an odorless acrylic is called the _____.

75. This layer is removed once the product _____ by using _____, _____, or a _____ product. It can also be _____.

76. To avoid skin contact, use a _____ when removing the _____.

77. If you choose to file away this layer _____.

78. Assume that you have just removed the nail forms. Use the letters A through G to show the correct order of the following steps:

   _____ Clean nails.

   _____ Buff the acrylic nail.

   _____ Apply polish.

   _____ Clear up your work area or table.

   _____ Apply oil to cuticles.

_____ Shape the free edge of the acrylic nail with a coarse or medium abrasive.

_____ Apply cream and perform massage.

79. **Matching.** *Match the terms on the left with correct descriptions, directions, or characteristics on the right.*

_____ 1. Push cuticle back.

_____ 2. Buff to remove shine.

_____ 3. Clean nails.

_____ 4. Apply nail dehydrator.

_____ 5. Apply tips.

_____ 6. Apply primer.

_____ 7. Prepare liquid and powder.

_____ 8. Dip brush into liquid and powder.

_____ 9. Place first bead.

_____ 10. Place second bead.

_____ 11. Use a gliding motion w/brush.

_____ 12. Shape nail.

_____ 13. Buff nail.

_____ 14. Apply nail oil.

_____ 15. Massage hands and arms.

_____ 16. Apply polish.

A. Wear plastic gloves and safety glasses

B. Dip briefly in liquid soap and water

C. Free edge down to nail plate

D. Rub into cuticles and surrounding skin

E. Use a light touch because the cuticle is dry

F. Pick up medium ball

G. Base coat, polish, topcoat

H. Attach plastic nails to client's natural nails

I. Used to smooth entire acrylic surface

J. Use 240-grit abrasives to remove natural oil

K. Use buffer to smooth entire acrylic surface

L. Use in small, separate containers

M. Place on nail's free edge

N. Use wooden pusher, cotton or spray to prevent bacteria growth

O. Use abrasive on the free edge.

P. Use hand cream or lotion

80. **Matching.** *Match the terms on the left with correct descriptions or definitions on the right.*

_____ 1. leads to polymerization

_____ 2. odorless acrylic (methacrylate) products

_____ 3. polymerization

_____ 4. chain reaction

_____ 5. ethyl methacrylate

_____ 6. catalyst

_____ 7. rebalancing

_____ 8. polymer

A. slightly different acrylic (methacrylate) products

B. curing, hardening

C. maintaining the beauty of the nail enhancement

D. made by combining monomers into long chains

E. used in monomer and polymer powder systems

F. made by combining monomer liquid/polymer powder

G. polymerization reaction

H. speeds up chemical reactions

I. initiator

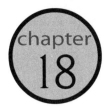

# UV Gels

## INTRODUCTION

1.  UV gels are cured with a _____. They are made from an _____ material.

2.  Most UV gels are made from _____. Newer UV gel technologies use _____.

3.  Match the following prefixes:

_____ 1. mono-          A. a few

_____ 2. oligo-          B. many

_____ 3. poly-           C. one

4.  UV gels rely on a related form of a monomer called an _____.

5.  In liquid and powder nail enhancements, _____ are liquids, and polymers are _____. _____ are somewhere in between.

6.  Oligomers usually have a _____, _____, _____ consistency.

7.  _____ is a special type of acrylate used in traditional UV gels.

8.  _____ are used in newer UV gel systems.

9.  UV gel nails have a high odor problem. True or false? _____

10. The UV lamp used to cure nails emits a special _____.

11. When applying a UV gel nail, you must expose the nail to _____ after _____ to the natural nail.

12. In addition to the materials required for a basic manicuring set-up, what other supplies and equipment will you need to do UV gels?

a. _____

b. _____

c. _____

d. _____

e. _____

f. _____

g. _____

13. UV light bulbs will stay blue for _____ , but after a few _____ of use they may produce too little UV light to properly _____ the enhancement.

14. When UV gel is exposed to UV light in its container, what happens? _____

15. The amount of electricity that a bulb consumes is called _____ .

16. Wattage indicates how much UV light is emitted. True or false? _____

17. Do all UV lamps emit the same amount of UV rays? _____
   _____

18. If you do not change UV bulbs on a regular basis, what do you risk?

   a. _____

   b. _____

19. You will have a much greater chance of success if you use the UV lamp _____
   _____ .

20. UV light bulbs have expired when they lose their blue color. True or false? _____
   _____

21. Depending on frequency of use, UV bulbs should be changed out _____ .

22. What is the purpose of UV gel primer? _____

23. What is the shelf life of nail adhesives? _____

24. Detail the UV gel application pre-service.

   a. Prepare your _____ with everything you need at your fingertips.

   b. Greet your client with a _____ .

   c. If this is your client's first appointment, a _____ should be prepared.

   d. If this is a return visit, perform client consultation, using the consultation form to record _____ .

25. You should always shape and shorten a nail tip prior to application when working with UV gel. Why? _____
   _____

26. Light-cured gel procedure. Using the list on top, fill in the bottom list with the application for light-cured gels in their correct order.

Apply base coat gel
Apply building UV gel
Apply hand lotion/Massage
Apply nail dehydrator
Apply nail oil
Apply Nail Polish
Apply Nail Tip (if desired)
Apply sealer or finisher UV gel

Check Nail contours
Clean nail enhancements
Clean Nails/Remove polish
Cure base coat gel
Cure builder UV gel
Prepare natural nail
Push back eponychium/remove cuticles

Remove dust
Remove inhibition layer
Remove inhibition layer
Remove oily shine

a. _____

b. _____

c. _____

d. _____

e. _____

f. _____

g. _____

h. _____

i. _____

j. _____

k. _____

l. _____

m. _____

n. _____

o. _____

p. _____

q. _____

r. _____

s. _____

27. Some manufacturers recommend that you apply UV gel to all _____ on each hand, and then _____.

28. When preparing the natural nails for a UV gel application, you should follow the _____ for _____.

29. Each layer of the UV gel should be cured for the time _____.

30. What could be the result of improperly curing the nails for too short a time?

    a. _____

    b. _____

31. Unlike acrylic nail enhancements, never use _____ with your brush. Instead,

_____ to create a _____.

32. Like odorless acrylic nail enhancements, an _____ is formed when UV gels harden. You can remove this layer with three of the following tools or products. *Circle the correct answers.*

    a. Acetone

    b. Benzoyl peroxide

    c. Alcohol

    d. Fine file (more than 240 grit)

    e. Buffer block

    f. Medium file (180 to 240 grit)

33. Your UV gel and brush should be kept away from _____, _____ and

_____ during the application process to prevent the product from prematurely

_____.

34. How do you know how long to cure your UV gel nail enhancements? _____

35. UV gels file very easily because _____.

36. Massaging nail oil onto the cuticle and skin _____.

37. Between each service, you should always _____ all used materials, and remove

_____ from your worktable to maintain the quality of

_____.

38. You must _____ UV gels every _____ weeks.

39. List the proper steps that you should do when removing UV gels. If the manufacturer recommends another way to remove UV gel nail enhancements, follow those directions.

    a. _____

    b. _____

    c. _____

    d. Gently buff the natural nail with a fine buffer _____.

    e. Condition skin with nail oil and lotion, or _____.

# The Creative Touch

## INTRODUCTION

1. Why should you develop nail art skills? _____.

2. To fulfill your potential as a nail artist, what should you do?

   a. Be _____.

   b. Expose yourself to all _____.

   c. _____ to your client.

   c. There is no such thing as an art mistake, only _____.

3. List the guiding business rules of nail art.

   a. Schedule _____ to perform the selected art.

   b. _____ your art.

   c. Be _____ priced.

   d. Invest in _____.

4. List six nail art services that you can perform on your clients' nails.

   a. _____

   b. _____

   c. _____

   d. _____

   e. _____

   f. _____

5. What should you always do before sealing your art? _____

6. What does floating the bead mean? _____

7. Why do you need a working knowledge of color theory to successfully perform nail art? _____

8. List the four color groups on the color wheel. Explain each group.

   a. _____

   b. _____

   c. _____

   d. _____

9. Red, yellow, and blue belong to which group of colors? _____

10. List the secondary colors you get when you mix equal parts of the following two colors:

    a. Red and yellow _____

    b. Yellow and blue _____

11. What is another name for tertiary colors? _____

## GEMS

12. How do you properly apply a gem?

    a. Apply topcoat _____ .

    b. Dampen the end of a wooden pusher with _____ .

    c. Pick up the gem by _____ .

    d. _____ .

    e. Apply a small amount of _____ .

    f. Finish with a _____ .

## FOILING

13. Foiling is available in a wide variety of colors and patterns. Name three of the most popular foil designs.

    _____

14. Describe Foiling Method #1.

    a. Polish the nail and allow it to completely dry.

    b. _____ .

    c. Select the foils you want to use, and _____ .

    d. _____ .

    e. Touch the backside of the foil to the surface of the nail, _____ .

    f. Do a light, quick _____ movement over the nail surface until _____

       _____

15. What should you take into consideration when choosing the polish color for foiling method #1?

    _____

16. How do you foil a nail? (Foiling method #2, opaque technique)

    a.–d. Follow steps a–d for Foiling method #1.

    e. _____

104

f. _____

17. Foiling method #2 provides a more _____ coverage of color.

18. As the sealer dries, you will see a _____.

## STRIPING TAPE

19. Striping tape has a _____ backing.

20. It is only applied to _____.

21. Although color selection of striping tape is generous, _____, _____, and _____ have been the most popular colors for years.

## GOLD LEAFING

22. Other names for gold leafing include _____ and _____.

23. Use _____ or the _____ when removing a gold leafing sheet from the packaging. Why? _____

24. How do you apply gold leafing?

    a. When the nail polish is completely dry, _____.

    b. _____

       Use _____ or a _____ for smaller pieces.

    c. _____.

    d. _____.

25. How do you create a nugget pattern? _____

## FREEHAND PAINTING

26. _____ is another term for freehand painting.

27. Brushes used in nail art vary from _____ and _____ bristle to _____ bristle.

28. What is the end of the brush called? _____

29. _____ have pointed tips; _____ have chiseled edges.

30. The _____ refers to the midsection of the brush.

31. A fluid stroke is accomplished by _____.

32. A spattered stroke is created by _____.

33. More _____ creates a wider stroke.

## MATCHING REVIEW

*Insert the correct word or term at the left of each definition.*

| flat brush | stylus | liner brush |
| striper brush | round brush | spotter brush |

34. _____ marbleizer used for creating polka dots, eyes, bubbles, and so on

35. _____ this brush holds a large amount of paint and gives long, fluid strokes

36. _____ has a tapered, pointed tip, and a large belly

37. _____ also known as a detailer; used for intricate, detail work

38. _____ good detail brush; used for line work, outlining, and lettering

39. _____ used to create long lines, and animal prints like zebra stripes

## USING AN AIRBRUSH FOR NAIL COLOR AND NAIL ART

40. How does an airbrush unit work? _____

41. Where does the air come from? _____

42. What are the best ways to practice doing airbrush nail art?

    a. Start by practicing on an _____.

    b. Practice spraying a _____.

    c. _____. To draw crisp lines, _____.

    d. _____.

    e. _____.

43. What do streaks or lines on the paper indicate when you are trying to paint an even area of color?

    _____

44. How do you remove accidental over-spray on the client's skin?

    a. _____

    b. _____

    c. _____

45. Airbrushing involves moving _____.

46. If you only move your wrist, what happens? _____.

47. Analogous colors are located _____ on the color wheel. They work beautifully when airbrushing _____.

48. What is the technique called that includes airbrushing two or more colors on the nail at the same time?

    _____

49. One of the most popular techniques used in airbrushing is the _____. Why? _____

    _____

50. Describe the principle that all airbrushes work on. (they combine air and paint to form an atomized spray). Describe how airbrushes differ.

    a. _____

    b. _____

    c. _____

51. Describe a gravity-fed airbrush system. _____.

52. Each airbrush has a small cone-shaped _____ that a tapered _____ fits into.

53. Explain why it is important to not touch the nail with the bristle of the airbrush. _____
_____

54. What is the most common air pressure used by nail technicians when airbrushing? _____
_____

55. List and describe the steps for an airbrushed version of a French manicure.

    a.   Apply a clear base coat to the nails.

    b.   _____

    c.   Optional: add a shimmer to the French manicure paint by misting a gold highlight or shimmer evenly over the French beige.

    d.   _____

    e.   Optional: mist the lunula slightly lighter than nail tip color.

    f.   Apply your nail paint bonder and let it dry _____; then apply _____
_____.

56. **Identification.** Using the letters **GL**, **G**, **T**, **F**, **A**, and **H** (defined below), match the correct characteristics listed with one form of nail art.

| Key: | Characteristics: |
|---|---|
| **GL** = gold leafing | _____ 1. comes in fragile sheets |
| **G** = gems | _____ 2. comes in rolls and is applied with an adhesive |
| **T** = striping tape | _____ 3. uses stencils |
| **F** = foil | _____ 4. gives sparkle and texture; is applied to a tacky topcoat |
| **A** = airbrushing | _____ 5. uses brush strokes to achieve a design |
| **H** = hand-painted (flat nail art) | _____ 6. comes in very thin rolls with adhesive backing |
| | _____ 7. can be reused if the silver backing is in place |
| | _____ 8. also known as nuggets |
| | _____ 9. shiny, colored side faces up |
| | _____ 10. paint is sprayed through a gun using a compressor |
| | _____ 11. applied to a dry, polished nail |
| | _____ 12. two colors can be used at the same time on one brush |

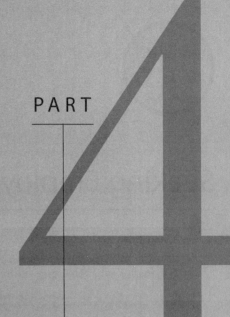

# BUSINESS SKILLS

PART

# Seeking Employment

## INTRODUCTION

1.  No matter what the state of the economy might be, there is always a demand for _____

    _____ .

2.  Name at least eight things that will help you pass your state board exam.

    a.  _____

    b.  _____

    c.  _____

    d.  _____

    e.  _____

    f.  _____

    g.  _____

    h.  _____

    i.  _____

    j.  _____

    k.  _____

    l.  _____

    m.  _____

3.  What steps should you take to ensure a successful ending on test day? List at least twelve things.

    a.  _____

    b.  _____

    c.  _____

    d.  _____

    e.  _____

    f.  _____

    g.  _____

        _____

    h.  _____

i. _____

j. _____

k. _____

l. _____

m. _____

n. _____

o. _____

p. _____

4. What is deductive reasoning? _____

5. List at least five test strategies involving deductive reasoning.

   a. _____

   b. _____

   c. _____

   d. _____

   e. _____

   f. _____

   _____

   g. _____

6. What is the best way to answer a true/false statement when you are not 100% sure of the answer?

   a. _____

   b. _____

   c. _____

7. How should you approach multiple-choice answers when you are not 100% sure of the answer?

   a. _____

   b. _____

   c. _____

   d. _____

   e. _____

   f. _____

   g. _____

   h. _____

   i. _____

   j. _____

8. How can you answer matching questions correctly?

   a. _____

   b. _____

9. What is the best way to approach essay questions?

a. _____

b. _____

c. _____

10. What is the best assurance you have to pass your state board test and become a licensed nail technician?

_____

11. List at least six things that you do can do pass your practical exam.

a. _____

b. _____

c. _____

d. _____

e. _____

f. _____

g. _____

h. _____

i. _____

## PREPARING FOR EMPLOYMENT

12. When looking for your first job, it is important to know what you want _____.

13. One way to help identify your practical skills and personal qualities is to complete a _____

_____.

14. What should you do about any areas that need more attention? _____

15. What are the key personal characteristics that will help you succeed?

a. _____

b. _____

c. _____

d. _____

e. _____

16. There are several different types of salons that you will want to consider before accepting your first job. Name these types and briefly describe each one.

a. _____

_____

b. _____

_____

c. _____

d. _____

_____

e. _____

f. _____

g. _____

_____

h. _____

_____

_____

17. What is the difference between a mid-priced, full-service salon and a high-end image salon or day spa?

_____

_____

_____

18. A written summary of your education and work experience is called what? _____

19. What is the average time spent reading a resume before the owner or manager decides whether to grant you an interview? _____

20. When writing your resume, you must _____ yourself in such a manner the reader will want to meet you.

21. Whenever possible, communicate your relevant skills and accomplishments in _____. Examples of this are:

_____

_____

_____

_____

_____

22. Name three things that you should not put on your resume.

a. _____

b. _____

c. _____

23. Define transferable skills. _____

24. List five things that you should include on your resume.

a. _____

b. _____

c. _____

d. _____

e. _____

25. What is an employment portfolio? _____
_____

26. You should start looking for your first salon position _____
_____.

27. Why should you begin networking as soon as possible? _____
_____

28. When you begin networking, your first contact should be _____.

29. What two things should you do in writing? _____
_____

30. List the seven most important things you should observe and rate when visiting a salon.

a. _____

b. _____

c. _____

d. _____

e. _____

f. _____

g. _____

h. _____

31. List twelve ways in which you can make a good impression at your first interview.

a. _____

b. _____

c. _____

d. _____

e. _____

f. _____

g. _____

h. _____

i. _____

j. _____

k. _____

l. _____

32.  What kinds of questions should you anticipate being asked? List them.

a. _____

b. _____

c. _____

d. _____

e. _____

f. _____

g. _____

h. _____

i. _____

j. _____

k. _____

l. _____

m. _____

n. _____

o. _____

p. _____

q. _____

r. _____

s. _____

33.  What questions should you prepare for your employment interview? List them.

a. _____

b. _____

c. _____

d. _____

e. _____

f. _____

g. _____

h. _____

i. _____

j. _____

k. _____

l. _____

34. List some legal questions that a potential employer can ask.

    a. _____

    b. _____

    c. _____

    d. _____

35. List some illegal questions that a potential employer cannot ask.

    a. _____

    b. _____

    c. _____

    d. _____

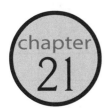

# On The Job

## INTRODUCTION

1. List the goals and rules that should guide you throughout your career:

   _____

   _____

2. Unlike the forgiving environment of school, in a salon situation you will be expected to

   _____ above your own. This means that

   _____.

3. List some personal habits that will allow you to provide excellent service.

   a. _____

   b. _____

   c. _____

   d. _____

   e. _____

   f. _____

   g. _____

4. A salon should be a team environment. True or false? _____

5. What does this mean? What do you have to do to be a team player?

   a. _____

   b. _____

   c. _____

   d. _____

   e. _____

   f. _____

   g. _____

   h. _____

6. What is a job description? _____

   _____

7. What are the three standard methods of compensation in a salon? Please explain.

a. _____

b. _____

_____

c. _____

_____

8. What is the best way to keep tabs on your progress in a salon setting? _____

_____

9. What is one of the best ways to improve your professional behavior? _____

_____

10. What two opportunities will you have to increase your income in a salon besides asking for a raise?

_____

11. What must you do to successfully recommend and sell products and services?

a. _____

b. _____

c. _____

d. _____

e. _____

f. _____

g. _____

h. _____

12. List the various reasons salon clients will buy salon products.

_____

_____

_____

13. List the marketing techniques you can use to keep your clients coming back for services.

a. _____

b. _____

c. _____

d. _____

e. _____

f. _____

g. _____

h. _____

i. _____

14. Always offer to _____ your clients. This will automatically improve your income because clients will _____ with their nails and visit you _____.

# The Salon Business

## INTRODUCTION

1.  Name two ways that you can go into business for yourself: ————————————————.

2.  What will you need to commit to in order to be a successful businessperson? ————————————————
    ———————————————————————————————————————————

3.  Over 50% of all licensed beauty professionals are now booth renters. True or false? ——————

4.  Many practitioners with large steady clienteles find that booth rental is a desirable situation. In general, a
    booth renter:

    a.  —————————————————————————————————————————

    b.  —————————————————————————————————————————

    c.  —————————————————————————————————————————

    d.  —————————————————————————————————————————

5.  When opening your own salon, you have more things to consider. Name some basic factors.

    a.  —————————————————————————————————

    b.  —————————————————————————————————

    c.  —————————————————————————————————

    d.  —————————————————————————————————

    e.  —————————————————————————————————

    f.  —————————————————————————————————

    g.  —————————————————————————————————

6.  What is a business plan? ——————————————————————————————————
    ———————————————————————————————————————————

7.  When preparing a business plan, a ————————————————— can be invaluable in helping
    you gather accurate financial information.

8.  There are three basic ways that you can own your own business. What are they?

    a.  ———————————————————————————

    b.  ———————————————————————————

    c.  ———————————————————————————

9. When purchasing an existing salon, what written documents must be provided to you before the close of sale?

a. _____

b. _____

c. _____

_____

d. _____

e. _____

f. _____

g. _____

_____

10. Your lease must specify clearly who owns what, and who is _____.

11. A simple and efficient _____ system is necessary to have a good business operation.

12. Record-keeping includes keeping track of salon inventory. List three things that an inventory system covers.

a. _____

b. _____

c. _____

13. When designing a new salon, _____ should be your top consideration.

14. Name some of the considerations when interviewing potential employees.

a. _____

b. _____

c. _____

d. _____

15. In terms of finances, your top priority is to _____.

16. If you do not see yourself as a natural manager, realize that you can _____.

17. First impressions count. What part of your salon should make a strong first impression?

_____

18. List the functions the receptionist handles in the salon:

a. _____

b. _____

c. _____

d. _____

e. _____

f. _____

19. A qualified receptionist handles the following responsibilities:

    a. _____ each client.

    b. Answering the _____.

    c. _____ appointments.

    d. Informing the _____ the client has _____.

    e. Preparing _____ for the staff.

    f. Recommending _____ to the client.

    g. _____ the reception area.

    h. Maintaining _____ and daily _____.

20. What information must be included for every salon appointment? _____

21. What is the best form of advertising? _____

## MATCHING REVIEW

*Insert the correct word or term to the left of each definition.*

| | | |
|---|---|---|
| booth rental | business plan | capital |
| consumption supplies | corporation | demographics |
| partnership | personnel | sole proprietor |
| retail supplies | booth renter | |

22. _____ an unincorporated business that is owned by a single individual

23. _____ a nail technician who pays a flat fee for use of a station

24. _____ a form of business that protects your personal assets

25. _____ information on the size, average income, and buying habits of consumers in a particular area or of a particular group

26. _____ also known as chair rental

27. _____ a plan that details the financial position of your business today and in the future

28. _____ available money for the operation and future growth of a business

29. _____ goods sold to clients

30. _____ goods needed for services and the daily running of the salon